Coping with Stom

DR TOM SMITH spent six years in general practice and seven years in medical research before taking up writing full-time in 1977. He wrote † octor Doctor' column in *The Guardian* Saturday magazine and the l columns in the *Sunday Mail*, the Bradford *Telegraph and Argus* and *ncashire Telegraph*. He has written three humorous books: *Doctor, ou got a minute?*, *A Seaside Practice*, and *Going Loco*, all published rt Books. His other books for Sheldon Press include *Heart Attacks: and Survive*; *Living with Alzheimer's Disease*; *Overcoming Back Pain*; with *Bowel Cancer*; *Coping with Heartburn and Reflux*; *Coping with ted Memory Loss*; *Skin Cancer: Prevent and Survive*; *How to Get the* D ' *Your Doctor*; *Coping with Kidney Disease*; *Osteoporosis: Prevent and* ' *bing Successfully with Prostate Cancer*; *Coping with Bronchitis and* *ema*; and *Living with Type 1 Diabetes*. He is married with two and five grandchildren.

Overcoming Common Problems Series

Selected titles

A full list of titles is available from Sheldon Press,
36 Causton Street, London SW1P 4ST and on our website at
www.sheldonpress.co.uk

101 Questions to Ask Your Doctor
Dr Tom Smith

Asperger Syndrome in Adults
Dr Ruth Searle

The Assertiveness Handbook
Mary Hartley

Assertiveness: Step by step
Dr Windy Dryden and Daniel Constantinou

Backache: What you need to know
Dr David Delvin

Birth Over 35
Sheila Kitzinger

Body Language: What you need to know
David Cohen

Bulimia, Binge-eating and their Treatment
Professor J. Hubert Lacey, Dr Bryony Bamford and
Amy Brown

The Cancer Survivor's Handbook
Dr Terry Priestman

The Chronic Pain Diet Book
Neville Shone

Cider Vinegar
Margaret Hills

Coeliac Disease: What you need to know
Alex Gazzola

Confidence Works
Gladeana McMahon

Coping Successfully with Pain
Neville Shone

Coping Successfully with Prostate Cancer
Dr Tom Smith

Coping Successfully with Psoriasis
Christine Craggs-Hinton

Coping Successfully with Ulcerative Colitis
Peter Cartwright

Coping Successfully with Varicose Veins
Christine Craggs-Hinton

Coping Successfully with Your Hiatus Hernia
Dr Tom Smith

Coping Successfully with Your Irritable Bowel
Rosemary Nicol

Coping When Your Child Has Cerebral Palsy
Jill Eckersley

Coping with Asthma in Adults
Mark Greener

Coping with Birth Trauma and Postnatal Depression
Lucy Jolin

Coping with Bowel Cancer
Dr Tom Smith

Coping with Bronchitis and Emphysema
Dr Tom Smith

Coping with Candida
Shirley Trickett

Coping with Chemotherapy
Dr Terry Priestman

Coping with Chronic Fatigue
Trudie Chalder

Coping with Coeliac Disease
Karen Brody

Coping with Diverticulitis
Peter Cartwright

Coping with Drug Problems in the Family
Lucy Jolin

Coping with Dyspraxia
Jill Eckersley

Coping with Early-onset Dementia
Jill Eckersley

Coping with Eating Disorders and Body Image
Christine Craggs-Hinton

Coping with Envy
Dr Windy Dryden

Coping with Epilepsy in Children and Young People
Susan Elliot-Wright

Coping with Gout
Christine Craggs-Hinton

Coping with Hay Fever
Christine Craggs-Hinton

Coping with Headaches and Migraine
Alison Frith

Coping with Heartburn and Reflux
Dr Tom Smith

Coping with Kidney Disease
Dr Tom Smith

Overcoming Common Problems Series

Overcoming Common Problems Series

Overcoming Common Problems

Coping with Stomach Ulcers

Second edition

DR TOM SMITH

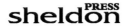

First published in Great Britain in 1996

Sheldon Press
36 Causton Street
London SW1P 4ST
www.sheldonpress.co.uk

Second edition published 2011

British Library Cataloguing-in-Publication Data
A catalogue record for this book is available from the British Library

ISBN 978-1-84709-206-9
eBook ISBN 978-1-84709-207-6

Typeset by Fakenham Prepress Solutions, Fakenham, Norfolk NR21 8NN
First printed in Great Britain by Ashford Colour Press
Subsequently digitally printed in Great Britain

Produced on paper from sustainable forests

Contents

For Laura

Introduction

One in every seven men in the UK has had a stomach or duodenal ulcer by the time he is 40. This figure seems huge, but in many developing countries the figure is much higher. Even in some countries in the Global North, like Japan, up to half of all men and around a quarter of all women have a history of ulcers. The real surprise, however, is that ulcers do not occur even more often. Because the miracle of the stomach is that its whole purpose is to digest food – which after all is made up of exactly the same materials as the stomach – without at the same time digesting itself. An ulcer arises when the stomach's protection from self-digestion breaks down.

Why ulcers occur, where they occur, how they affect you, and how they can be treated and prevented, is the subject of this book. It is meant for people with ulcers and their partners and families.

The first edition was written in 1992, at a time of completely new thinking among doctors about the causes and treatment of ulcers. Much of the time-honoured advice about ulcers had been shown to be completely wrong. For example, eating particular foods does not cause ulcers – a normal stomach can cope well with curries or fries – and turning to a bland milky diet does not cure them. In fact it can make you even more ill.

There is little evidence that stress is a major cause of ulcers or that changing your lifestyle helps much once you have acquired an ulcer.

Before the 1990s no doctor would have considered that ulcers might be caused by an infection: the very idea would have been laughed at. Students suggesting such a thing would have been failed. It was thought that the stomach digestive juice was too acidic for any germ to survive in it. Yet now, duodenal ulcer, in particular, can be cured and its recurrence prevented not by prescribing the classical drugs to neutralize acidity, but by treating it as an infection with a cocktail of antibacterial drugs.

This followed the discovery that deep in the lining of the stomach in many people with ulcers there is a thriving colony of bacteria called *Helicobacter pylori*. This germ is unique, as far as we know, to the human gut. Its link with ulcers was sprung upon doctors in the early 1980s, but it took more than a decade for it to be accepted. One chapter of this book is devoted to *Helicobacter* and its treatment.

But before *Helicobacter* came 'H_2 antagonists'. These drugs – the first were cimetidine and ranitidine (Tagamet and Zantac) – are now household names. They won a Nobel Prize for the researchers who discovered them and have made billions of pounds for the pharmaceutical companies marketing them. And they revolutionized the treatment of ulcers. With them, the need to operate on ulcerated stomachs virtually disappeared overnight. People could at last live with their illness – although the drugs had to be continued for perhaps years to avoid recurrences.

The story of H_2 antagonists and their successors the 'proton pump inhibitors', the first of which was omeprazole (Losec), is also told in the chapters on treatment.

However, drugs are not the only aspect of management of ulcers. They must be taken along with a reappraisal of your lifestyle. Lifestyle changes alone may not help, but in combination with active antiulcer treatment they can greatly improve your quality of life. The aim of this book is to do just that – to improve the quality of life for all people with ulcers, and their sometimes equally suffering carers!

1

Ulcers, indigestion and dyspepsia: how to tell them apart

The crucial symptom of an ulcer is pain. It can be just a discomfort to some, and a severe, crippling, work-stopping pain to others, and it can be of any severity between these two extremes.

The pain is usually in the pit of the stomach, the depression in the abdomen just below the breastbone, in the centre. However, it can also bore into the back, or spread further down the abdomen to the navel. Pain below the navel is almost certainly not due to an ulcer.

Some describe the pain as a gnawing sensation, which is interesting, as very few people have ever actually been gnawed! Doctors hearing that description are quickly alerted to the possibility of an ulcer. Others describe the pain as like toothache, and still others as a burning sensation.

A pain that virtually clinches the diagnosis of ulcer, almost without the need to do further tests, is one that wakens you around 2.00 a.m. It is relieved quickly by a drink of milk or an antacid preparation – anything from sodium bicarbonate to one of the hundreds of complicated aluminium- or magnesium-containing mixtures available from your pharmacy. I have known people with an ulcer to keep a glass of beer beside their bed as their most effective and immediate relief, which suggests that for some of them the pain may be 'washed away' purely by the diluting action of water as effectively as it is neutralized by an antacid. There is anecdotal evidence (from a doctor who treated his fellow political prisoners) that water (all he could give them) did ease their ulcer symptoms, and that drinking it before and after their less than nutritious meals helped to keep them clear of further pain.

Some people find that vomiting relieves the pain. The material they bring up is often acidic, so it is sour-tasting, and is usually bile-stained (green or yellow). It used to be thought that this was a sign

1

of an ulcer in the duodenum (see Chapter 2), but it can occur with both stomach and duodenal ulcers.

The pain often relates to eating, but in different ways in different people. For a very few people the act of eating brings on almost immediate pain. Frankly, this is more commonly a sign of nervous dyspepsia (explained below) than of ulcer, although it may, in a few people, denote a stomach (gastric) ulcer.

It is much more common for ulcer pain to start 2–3 hours after a meal, when the stomach is empty, and for it to be relieved by another snack. Many ulcer-prone people, snacking like this for years, put on a lot of weight as a result.

For some people the pain is a daily event. It is never there on waking or before breakfast, but starts around noon and gradually worsens throughout the day, being worse in the evening. It is also relieved by antacids or food, and people with this type of pain always carry antacid tablets around with them, chewing them several times a day. If you are into this daily habit you should seek your doctor's advice.

Ulcer symptoms of all types are 'periodic' in that they may bother people for days or even a few weeks at a time, then disappear, perhaps for months or a year or two. Many people with an ulcer follow this pattern throughout their adult lives, and can give no obvious reason for the relapsing/improving pattern of symptoms.

An extra symptom, apart from the pain, that signifies probable ulcer disease is waterbrash. This is a sudden filling of the mouth with saliva. It goes along with heartburn, a hot, burning feeling in the centre of the chest behind the breastbone. Waterbrash and heartburn are also signs of hiatus hernia, in which there is ulceration of the lower oesophagus (see Chapter 2), and this, too, needs to be taken into account when the diagnosis is made.

'Dyspepsia' or 'indigestion'

Here, something must be said about 'dyspepsia' or 'indigestion'. Many people label their symptoms with one of these words. Medically they are meaningless, and have more to do with the long history of patent medicine advertising than medical accuracy. People complaining of dyspepsia or indigestion usually describe their pain as hot, burning or bloating, rather than gnawing or dull and aching.

Dyspepsia is commonly thought of as pain or discomfort in the upper abdomen or the centre of the chest linked to eating. Dyspeptic and ulcer pains differ, therefore, in their timing and severity. Untreated ulcer pain lasts at the same level of intensity for an hour or more. Dyspepsia is sharper and shorter, coming in spasms. Both must be differentiated from colic, in which the pain shoots to a climax, then dies away, only to reappear a few minutes later, and to continue in cycles of painful and pain-free periods.

Colic can arise from the gall bladder and bile ducts or the large bowel. Gall bladder colic tends to be felt in the upper right quarter of the abdomen, just below the ribs. It may occur in the midline, where ulcer pain is felt, but it is never left-sided. Bowel colic is mainly in the left lower abdomen, below the navel. Pain felt only below the navel is likely to come from bowel or bladder irritation, and is almost never due to peptic ulcer.

Symptoms of dyspepsia or indigestion are *not* by themselves signs of ulcers. They are much more likely to be the result of a 'nervous gut', in which the mechanisms, nervous and hormonal, controlling the process of digestion throughout the gut are disturbed.

People with dyspepsia, for example, often complain of 'acidity', despite the fact that, when their stomach juices are examined, their acid level is normal or even below normal. Television advertisements featuring remedies for 'acid indigestion' can be most misleading. People who cannot tolerate 'acid' foods such as oranges or orange juice have to come to terms with the unpalatable fact (to them) that their own stomach juices are far more acid than the offending food.

Others claim that a particular food is 'indigestible' or 'disagrees' with them. Sadly, when they agree to investigation of their stomach juices, it is proved time and again that the suspect food is digested as easily and with as little reaction as any other. When the food (fried fatty foods and cheeses are good examples) is given by gastric tube, so that it is not tasted and is unknown to the person taking it, there is no reaction and it is treated by the stomach in exactly the same way as other digestible foods!

Food allergies as a cause of indigestion or dyspepsia must also be very much rarer than is claimed. Researchers studying the processes going on in the stomach, duodenum and the rest of the gut have shown that the so-called allergenic foods are digested as easily as any other and cause no abnormal reaction within the stomach. All the evidence points to the fact that indigestion due to food allergy is more in the mind than in the stomach. One exception, and that is rare, is cow's milk allergy in small children. This causes diarrhoea rather than indigestion.

Diseases that are truly caused by intolerance to particular foods include coeliac disease, which is a reaction to gluten, a component of many flours and grains. This, too, causes diarrhoea and weight loss rather than dyspepsia or indigestion. It affects the small bowel, rather than the stomach or duodenum.

Sorting out the cause of your pain

By the time you have read this far you will have recognized that you cannot diagnose the source of any stomach pain just from the symptoms alone. Stomach pains vary in their quality, their severity, their timing, their position, their relation with food and sleep, and in the actions that bring them on (if any).

However, there are some guidelines that help to sort out ulcer symptoms from those due to other causes. They are not hard and fast, but if you have some of the pointers to ulcer they should make you think twice about treating yourself for indigestion or dyspepsia and encourage you to go to your doctor for examination and tests.

Pointers towards ulcer include:

- Pain in the pit of the stomach, not far to either side, above the navel, gnawing or boring and not necessarily severe, that persists for an hour or more and fluctuates a little without being colicky.
- If the area of pain is so localized that you can point to it with one finger consistently, it is more than likely to be ulcer pain.
- Pain that starts when you are hungry, rather than immediately after food, or wakes you up at night. It may get worse gradually during the day. It is *eased* by food, milk or antacids, not worsened by them.

- It can be so frequent that it makes you snack between meals (to stop it), so that you put on weight, rather than lose it.
- It can appear for a few days at a time, then disappear for weeks, months or even years before it recurs.
- Even when there is ulcer pain there is no tenderness when the doctor presses firmly down on the painful area. The exception to this is when there are complications, which are described below.

Pointers towards nervous dyspepsia include:

- Pain in the pit of the stomach, but usually also elsewhere in the abdomen, to the left or right, or below. It starts immediately after eating, sometimes a specific food to which the person feels sensitive. It is not eased particularly well by antacids or milk, and certainly not by more food.
- It is usually a sharp pain, like a burning sensation: it is often linked with a bloating feeling and with sickness. It is not closely defined – you are most likely to use several fingers to indicate a vague, relatively wide area of upper abdomen as the area of discomfort.
- It is not a hunger pain and does not wake you up at night. In fact you may not get to sleep easily because of your nervousness and anxiety.
- Your appetite seems normal until you start to eat, then after a mouthful or two you feel too full and your appetite disappears completely. You begin eating, then stop, and leave much of the food on your plate.
- You are troubled by belching. The wind is odourless, or smells of the food you have just eaten. This type of wind is swallowed air: people with nervous dyspepsia are constantly swallowing air without being aware of it, and what goes down has to come up again! Sometimes the wind travels all the way through the gut to give flatulence. Neither belching nor flatulence is a sign of ulcer.
- As you eat three meals a day you tend to blame your pain on any food you may have eaten up to several days beforehand, quite erroneously.
- Nervous dyspepsia is often associated with some tenderness in the general area of the stomach. If the patient reacts with tenderness to the doctor's examination, without there being other signs

of complications, this is a strong sign that there is *no* ulcer, and that the diagnosis is dyspepsia.

Two distinguished gastroenterologists, Elwyn Elias and Clifford Hawkins (I'm proud to say one of my teachers at medical school), describe the typical symptoms of nervous dyspepsia as follows:

> Sensitivity to food occurs and patients become introspective about eating, finding that various, and in some cases every, type of food and drink causes symptoms. Even the smell of food may start trouble. One patient stated that she knew by telepathy whether food was about even if she could not see or smell it. Another was able to enjoy New Zealand lamb but English lamb made her ill for days afterwards. No one's stomach has this remarkable power of discrimination.

Other symptoms of nervous dyspepsia include nausea and dislike of anything tight around the waist. Dyspeptics may complain of heartburn, but it is not like the heartburn of ulcer, which lasts only a few minutes. Nervous dyspeptic heartburn lasts hours, and even a whole day.

Finally, nervous dyspeptics are often unwell in ways unrelated to the stomach and digestion. Their complaints can include tiredness, sleeplessness, dizziness, headache, depression and sexual difficulties. Most people with an ulcer are fit, except for their ulcer symptoms.

Exceptions to the ulcer rules

Of course, there are always exceptions to any statement on health matters. Eating fats does cause indigestion in some people with ulcers. A sudden aversion to fatty food such as bacon and eggs or chocolate can be a first sign of duodenal ulcer. Why this should be is obscure, because fats stimulate neither acidity nor excess gut activity – both of which have been thought to cause ulcers.

In some people with stomach (gastric) rather than duodenal ulcer (see Chapter 2 for the difference), the pain starts soon after food, so that it can mimic dyspepsia on that point alone. However, it still has all the other characteristics of ulcer pain, rather than of nervous dyspepsia.

If ulcer pain does deviate from the midline to one or other side, it is likely to be to the left with gastric ulcers and to the right with duodenal ulcers, but the deviation is never more than 2–5 cm. Ulcers in the lower end of the oesophagus, associated with hiatus hernia (see Chapter 2), give pain in the centre of the chest and can mimic angina due to heart disease. Bending over or lying flat can trigger this type of pain, and it can lead to persistent heartburn. It differs from angina (and from dyspeptic heartburn) in that antacids quickly relieve it.

Warning signs: the complicated ulcer

In itself, peptic ulcer is not a fatal disease. Most people live with their ulcers for years, and never experience more than discomfort and occasional periods of pain that can be managed by medicines. However, life-threatening complications *can* arise, and you must know how to recognize them, so that if they occur you can see your doctor about them as soon as possible.

Ulcers can perforate, bleed and cause obstruction.

Perforation

In perforation, the ulcer has penetrated through the wall of the stomach or duodenum, allowing digestive juices to pass outside the gut into the surrounding peritoneal cavity. The result is peritonitis: people whose ulcers have perforated must be admitted very quickly to hospital, where they will need emergency surgery.

The symptoms of perforation start suddenly, so much so that patients can pinpoint its exact time. The pain is much more severe than usual, forcing you to stop whatever you are doing and lie down. Any movement makes the pain worse. It can bore into the back or into a shoulder tip, depending on whether the gastric juice flows back towards the pancreas or up towards the diaphragm. It can even cause pain in the lower half of the abdomen, simulating appendicitis or a pelvic infection.

Normally the abdomen feels soft, but immediately after a perforation the abdominal muscles become rigid and board-like. It can be difficult to breathe, as the inflammation spreads to the diaphragm and the lower part of the lungs. During this initial period you are pale, sweaty and have a fast pulse.

Between 1 and 4 hours after the perforation there is a brief period when you feel better, the pain is less and if you have not called the doctor by this time you may be tempted not to do so. That is the big mistake, as this is the beginning of generalized peritonitis, leading to shock, infection and death if it is untreated.

Bleeding

Bleeding is much less dramatic, but can be as lethal as perforation if ignored or undiagnosed. It occurs when the ulcer erodes into an artery in the stomach or duodenal wall. However, bleeding by itself does not cause pain. Instead, it shows itself in one of two ways – depending on whether the loss of blood is sudden and large or gradual and persistent.

In the first case the bleeding causes a sudden drop in blood pressure, with fainting and shock. There may be vomiting of material that looks like coffee grounds (haematemesis), which is blood altered in appearance by contact with stomach acid and other digestive juices. Urgent admission to hospital is needed to replace the lost blood, and for the bleeding to be stopped. Until recently that needed surgery, but modern drug treatment has been very successful in returning many patients to normal without the need for an operation.

More often, bleeding does not cause a sudden crisis but is measured in terms of a few millilitres a day. Over weeks and months the blood loss adds up, so that you become wan and pale. The symptoms bringing you to the doctor may not appear at all relevant to the stomach or duodenum: they may simply be the usual symptoms of anaemia – mainly tiredness, weakness and breathlessness on the slightest exertion. Blood tests will confirm the loss of blood, and tests for blood in the stools will be positive. The stools may be black and tarry (melaena) if more than 10 ml blood is being lost per day, but smaller losses than this are identified from specific tests of stool samples and do not appear obvious in your stools. Losses of more than 5 ml blood per day over long periods lead to anaemia.

Obstruction

The crucial symptom in obstruction due to ulcer is vomiting. The obstruction occurs because scarring at the site of a long-standing ulcer (usually around the pylorus – the junction between the stomach and the duodenum – see Chapter 2), has caused narrowing of the gut at that point, and food can no longer pass through it. This condition is called pyloric stenosis.

In obstruction, the vomit contains considerable amounts of fluid, mainly gastric juice, along with undigested food that is free of bile (which cannot pass upwards past the obstruction from the duodenum into the stomach). Often the patient belches a lot of foul-smelling wind. If there is pain, it is usually an upper abdominal cramp or feelings of fullness and bloating in the upper abdomen, which are eased by vomiting.

With obstruction, there is loss of appetite with considerable and rapid weight loss. Most obstructed patients are constipated, although around a quarter of them have diarrhoea. In contrast to patients with bleeding, who are often very agitated, obstruction leaves people lethargic and weak because of dehydration.

Could my ulcer be malignant?

Benign peptic ulcers do not become malignant, so that people who have had ulcer symptoms or dyspepsia for years and whose symptoms have not changed need not fear that they have cancer. However, malignancies can arise in people who have had ulcers, and it is important to recognize the usual warning signs.

Such cancers are exclusive to the stomach: they are virtually unknown in the duodenum. The cardinal signs are loss of appetite (anorexia), vague discomfort and fullness in the pit of the stomach, loss of energy and loss of weight. The stools may change in character, so that you may become constipated for the first time or start to pass looser stools than you are used to. If there is pain it is of the boring type, rather than the burning type of dyspepsia. It is often felt through to the back.

Stomach cancers can cause bleeding, difficulty in swallowing, vomiting, perforation and obstruction, so they can present a picture just like a complicated ulcer. Occasionally, people come to their doctor with a mass in their stomach that they have found by chance, and has caused absolutely no symptoms.

Obviously, the earlier a cancer is detected the better the chance of survival, so if you find any of the above symptoms, please see your doctor at once. It is still odds on that you have a benign ulcer – ulcers outnumber cancers by around 20:1 – but you must rule out a tumour to give yourself the best chance of cure.

Is my ulcer gastric or duodenal?

Doctors used to try to pinpoint the site of an ulcer from the symptoms alone. It is only recently that we have had to admit that this is not only very difficult – duodenal and stomach ulcers give rise to similar symptoms – but it is not even very useful, as the treatment is often the same, regardless of the ulcer site.

In Britain, duodenal ulcers are around four to five times more common than gastric ulcers, the ratio varying from 3:1 in the South East to 9:1 in Scotland. In other countries there are very different figures, with gastric ulcers predominating in Japan, for example. People with blood group O are 40 per cent more likely to develop duodenal ulcer and 20 per cent more likely to develop gastric ulcer than people with blood groups A, B and AB. Why this should be is unclear: it may be that the blood group genes also strongly influence the character of the mucus that protects the stomach and duodenum from ulceration (see Chapter 2). On the other hand, people with gastric cancer are more likely to possess blood group A than O.

Another major difference between gastric and duodenal ulcers is the level of acid in the stomach. Acid levels are low and sometimes even absent in gastric ulcer, but much higher than normal in duodenal ulcer. However, some people with gastric ulcer have very high acid levels: they have Zollinger–Ellison syndrome, a condition explained in Chapter 2.

Sex differences

There is also a difference between the sexes. A peptic ulcer, and especially duodenal ulcer, is much more common in men than in women. Until puberty ulcers are rare, but they are equally divided between boys and girls. An ulcer should be one of the diagnoses considered in a child who repeatedly wakes up in the early hours with tummy pains.

Women appear to be protected against ulcers by their hormones, and in those women who do develop them, they are much less severe. Pregnancy relieves ulcer symptoms. There is no difference between the sexes in stomach acid secretion, and neither pregnancy nor hormone treatment reduces acid secretion. All this evidence suggests, therefore, that acid is only part of the ulcer story, and this is explained in the next chapter.

2

Normal digestion: and what goes wrong in ulcers

To understand ulcer disease we need to know about the relationship between the oesophagus, the stomach and the duodenum and the mechanisms of digestion (see Figure 1).

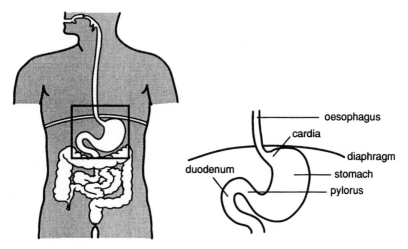

Figure 1

The oesophagus

The oesophagus is a muscular tube deep in the centre of the chest, leading from the throat to the stomach. We start to swallow food and drink by consciously contracting the muscles in our throat, but the process continues quite unconsciously with muscular contractions that ripple down our oesophagus towards the stomach. Gravity plays no part in swallowing: you can drink perfectly satisfactorily when standing on your head. The oesophagus sees to it that the fluid travels in the right direction, even if it is in an upward direction, towards the stomach!

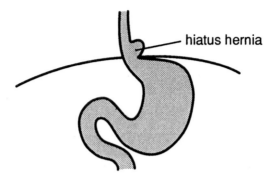

hiatus hernia

Figure 2a

The food enters the stomach from the oesophagus through a gap in the diaphragm, the sheet of muscle that separates the contents of the chest from the contents of the abdomen. This gap is effectively a ring of muscle, known as the cardia, which contracts neatly around the entrance of the stomach and prevents any reverse flow of the contents of the stomach back into the oesophagus.

Take away this valve mechanism, and acid and pepsin (a protein-digesting enzyme) from the stomach will come into contact with the delicate lining of the oesophagus and erode it, causing ulceration. This is what happens in hiatus hernia (see Figure 2a).

In hiatus hernia, a portion of the stomach is out of position, above the diaphragm. This allows backflow of digestive juices from the stomach into the oesophagus which, unlike the stomach, is not protected against them. The backward flow is obviously greater if you are bending over or lying flat, and reduced considerably by keeping upright, which is why you are advised to keep upright during the day and to sleep on three or four pillows at night if you have a hiatus hernia. The irritation of the lower end of the oesophagus caused by backward flow of acid and pepsin is described as oesophagitis.

The stomach

The stomach is an expandable bag, within which food entering from the oesophagus is thoroughly mixed with the digestive juices hydrochloric acid and pepsin. The wall of the stomach therefore has to be muscular, to produce the mixing; be lined with cells

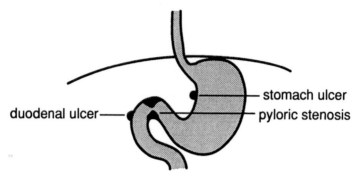

duodenal ulcer —————

stomach ulcer

pyloric stenosis

Figure 2b

secreting the gastric juices; and be fitted with some form of protection against self-digestion by the same juices.

Looked at through an endoscope (a flexible fibre-optic tube), the stomach lining is orange-red and glistens from a coating of mucus. There are thick folds in the wall that smooth out when it is filled with food or fluid. The muscle wall of the stomach is in constant movement, to churn up the food and to ensure it passes slowly on towards the exit from the stomach, the pylorus, and into the duodenum.

The lining of the stomach contains the cells that secrete the gastric juices that start off the process of digestion. Many of them are zymogen cells that secrete the enzyme pepsinogen, which on contact with acid becomes pepsin. Pepsin starts off the process of digesting the proteins in our food – meat, fish and vegetable proteins alike. Without the acid, pepsin does not form from pepsinogen, and does not act upon the protein.

Alongside the zymogen cells are the parietal or oxyntic cells that secrete hydrochloric acid. This is strong hydrochloric acid, around pH1, a concentration that would burn if spilled on your skin. People vary in the number of parietal cells they possess: they are far more numerous than normal in many people with duodenal ulcer – and often almost absent in people with gastric ulcer.

The other cells vital to a normal stomach wall are mucus-secreting goblet cells. The sticky mucus adheres to the stomach wall surface, forming a barrier to acid attack. It also contains bicarbonate, an alkali that neutralizes the acid and stops the activity of pepsin, a double action that gives extra protection to the stomach wall.

The stomach is always, therefore, on a knife edge. On the one hand it must produce enough acid and pepsin to start the process of digestion. On the other it must produce enough mucus and bicarbonate to prevent its own acid and pepsin from digesting itself. Anything that breaks down the mucus/bicarbonate protection allows access of acid and pepsin to the stomach lining, which then starts to be digested like any item of food. This area of self-digestion is an ulcer (see Figure 2b).

The stomach is protected from this process by a hugely sophisticated series of nerve and chemical 'messages' that start even before food enters the stomach. For example, in between meals stomach activity is relatively quiet. Acid and pepsin secretion is minimal, and may even be absent. This is particularly true during sleep: in people without ulcers there is a nightly fall in stomach secretion of acid and pepsin, so that digestion slows and the stomach rests.

The process of activating the mechanisms of digestion in the stomach starts with hunger and the sight and smell of food. This first of all triggers release of saliva into the mouth, then kick-starts the secretions in the stomach. The latter arise from stimulation of the vagus nerve, which runs from the brain directly to the stomach wall. Stimulation of the vagus activates the cells secreting all the components – acid, pepsinogen, mucus and bicarbonate – needed for digestion and protection.

As the food enters the stomach from the oesophagus, its contact with the lower half of the stomach reinforces the digestive process: it causes the lining cells there to release into the bloodstream the hormone gastrin, which in turn causes the other stomach lining cells to release yet more acid and pepsin. In a short third phase, as the partly digested food begins to reach the duodenum, beyond the stomach, further gastrin is released by duodenal lining cells. This stimulates yet more acid and pepsin release by the stomach lining cells.

At first the stomach acts as a reservoir, keeping the food inside itself to ensure that mixing between food and digestive juice is thorough. Then, slowly, the mixture is passed onwards to the exit, to the pylorus and duodenum, so that between 2 and 5 per cent of the gastric contents, by this time a liquid, is delivered to the duodenum each minute. The stomach is in effect a rhythmic pump, delivering a small proportion of its contents at a fixed rate through the pylorus after each meal, until it is empty.

The speed of stomach emptying depends on the type of food inside it. Sugars and starches speed up emptying, fats slow it down. This may be one reason for the common feeling that Chinese meals, which are mainly starch, only fill you up for a short time, while fish and chips, largely fat, are more satisfying for longer. Fluids leave the stomach faster than solids, which may explain why drinkers can take in many pints at a time and why, if they want to cut down, they should eat along with their drinking.

Emotions also alter gastric emptying. Sadness slows it down, anger speeds it up; perhaps this is why we tend to lose our appetite when we are depressed and why we can be ravenous when agitated and angry.

Gastric emptying is also faster in people with duodenal ulcers, except where the ulcers have caused scarring to the pylorus or the antrum (the last part of the stomach) that holds up the smooth onward passage of the mixture of food and digestive juice. The scarring can cause narrowing, or stenosis, at the pylorus (see Figure 2b). Gastric emptying is normal in people with gastric ulcers.

The pylorus, like the cardia at the entry to the stomach from the oesophagus, works like a valve. Muscles in the pyloric wall contract to stop the contents travelling back into the stomach from the duodenum beyond.

The duodenum

Beyond the pylorus, the environment in the duodenum is very different from that in the stomach. As the stomach contents become more and more acid, and sugars and fats start to enter the duodenum in greater quantity, the signals change, so that the stomach receives the message to stop secreting acid and the duodenum is triggered to deliver the hormone secretin into the bloodstream. The target of secretin is the pancreas, which on receiving its message releases its alkaline digestive juices into the duodenum. These neutralize any remaining acid and inactivate any remaining pepsin from the stomach. They are helped by the bile that is at the same time being squirted into the duodenum from the liver.

From the final part of the duodenum onwards, the contents of the intestine are alkaline and not acid, and the possibility of peptic ulcer occurring lower down in the gut, in the rest of the small intestine, is no longer a problem.

How it can all go wrong

By now, the complexity of the system regulating the balance between digestion and protection should be obvious – and so should the fact that there are many areas within the system in which things can go wrong. There may be excessive acid/pepsin secretion. The mucous resistance to acid and pepsin attack may become deficient. Either side of the acid/pepsin:mucus/bicarbonate equation may be altered by drugs or infection.

Popular myths about the causes of peptic ulcer need to be exploded. For example, irregular meals, different foods, poor dentition, alcohol and smoking have all been suggested in the past as causes of ulcer: none have been proven. Smoking may worsen symptoms in an already established ulcer, but does not initiate the change. Alcohol may induce gastritis – an irritation of the whole stomach lining – but it does not cause gastric or duodenal ulcer by itself. However, like smoking, it can worsen an already established ulcer.

Excessive acid and pepsin

For many people with duodenal ulcer the fault seems to lie in an excess of parietal cells, so that they produce just too much acid. For others the problem is that they do not have the night-time fall in acid production, so that during the hours of sleep, acid is constantly dripping from the stomach into the duodenum without the neutralizing effect of food or pancreatic juices. This helps to explain why so many people with an ulcer are wakened by pain in the night.

Excess acid is taken to extremes in Zollinger–Ellison syndrome. People with Zollinger–Ellison have tumours (usually benign) in their pancreas that secrete large amounts of gastrin into the bloodstream. The stomach responds to the gastrin by secreting a huge amount of acid, which overcomes the mucus and bicarbonate protection. Zollinger–Ellison syndrome was until recently a life-threatening disease, causing very severe stomach and duodenal ulcers with a very high risk of perforation and bleeding. As the pancreatic tumours are very difficult to detect or remove, the only treatment used to be complete removal of the stomach; thankfully we now have drugs to neutralize the gastrin effect. This is explained in more detail in the chapter on drug treatments.

A major symptom of Zollinger–Ellison syndrome is diarrhoea, which may start before the ulcer symptoms. This is because so much acid is produced by the stomach and escapes into the duodenum that it cannot be neutralized there by the alkaline pancreatic juices or bile. This makes the contents of the small intestine beyond the duodenum acid, rather than alkaline, and the whole fluid balance within the gut is disturbed – hence the diarrhoea. A combination of diarrhoea and severe ulcer symptoms should always raise the suspicion of Zollinger–Ellison syndrome, but it may still be the result of extreme excess of acid secretion by a larger than normal number of parietal cells in the stomach.

Defective protection

Most people with gastric ulcers and a few with duodenal ulcers have normal acid and pepsin levels in their stomachs. In fact, many people with gastric ulcer have very low acid levels. So other mechanisms than simply excess acid must be at work in many people. The obvious culprit is the mucosal protection. We know that the mucus loses its protective effect against acid in the later stages of severe illnesses. Patients near death develop multiple erosions of the stomach and duodenum that are due to loss of mucus, and not to excess acid or pepsin. These 'stress ulcers' are nevertheless not typical of peptic ulcer, where there is no consistent evidence of problems with the mucus itself.

The mucus layer can be broken down, however, by certain chemical substances, such as drugs or alcohol, or even by the bile acids produced from the patient's own liver.

It is important at this point to understand the role of aspirin and other antirheumatic and antiarthritic drugs in damaging this ulcer-preventing system. The secretion of the mucus and its bicarbonate content is promoted by a substance called prostaglandin E_2, which forms in the stomach wall. Prostaglandins also feature elsewhere in the body – particularly in joints – as the chemicals released in the perception of pain and inflammation. Aspirin and all other anti-inflammatory drugs like it, such as ibuprofen, indometacin and naproxen (non-steroidal anti-inflammatory drugs; NSAIDs), ease pain by preventing the formation of prostaglandins.

Counteracting prostaglandins is good for easing the pain of inflamed joints but is completely wrong in the stomach, because without prostaglandin secretion the mucus protection is reduced or lost. The result is multiple small erosions in the stomach, and the symptoms of stomach ulcer. People with an ulcer should there-fore avoid taking drugs that they know will upset their stomachs. Many manufacturers now offer these drugs in formulations such as capsules or even suppositories designed not to irritate the stomach, so that if this is part of your problem you may be able to switch to one that suits you better.

Another way manufacturers tried to avoid causing ulcers in people who must take regular NSAIDs was to combine them with a form of prostaglandin E_2, misoprostol. After the first decade of its use along with the NSAIDs diclofenac and naproxen the combina-tion is well accepted, but at times it does not seem to work as well as the theory suggests. Many people with chronic joint pains (as in rheumatoid arthritis) need a higher dose of misoprostol than the combined drug contains.

Corticosteroid drugs (steroids) such as prednisolone or cortisone taken by mouth for long periods can also cause chronic ulcers in the stomach and duodenum, probably by damaging the mucus protection. However, the dose needed to produce an ulcer is large, usually above 15 mg prednisolone per day. This high dose is unusual nowadays; for example, in asthma most steroids are now given in very much smaller doses by inhalation directly into the lungs, and in arthritis newer drugs have allowed the long-term dose of steroid to be reduced to around 2.5 or 5 mg per day or on alternate days.

Strong alcohol also destroys the mucosal protection, so that if you are prone to ulcers you should avoid it. Saving alcohol such as wine for meal times, and doing without neat spirits, is a good rule.

Nicotine from smoking probably has a similar destructive effect on the gastric mucus. Certainly, stopping smoking is at least as good as long-term antiulcer treatment in preventing relapses of ulcer symptoms.

Helicobacter pylori: gastritis and ulcer linked

No explanation of how ulcers are formed could now be complete without bringing in *Helicobacter pylori*. This is a bacterium found only in the stomach, closely related with – in fact stuck to – the mucosa, the lining layer of cells. It has been very positively linked with the initiation and recurrence of duodenal ulcer, and its eradication with drugs relieves ulcer symptoms. How it causes ulcers is not yet completely clear, but it is important enough for it to take up the whole of the next chapter of this book.

3

Enter the villain: *Helicobacter pylori*

In April 1982, Dr B. J. Marshall, a young hospital physician training in gastroenterology at the Royal Perth Hospital, Western Australia, left a specimen taken from the stomach of an ulcer patient incubating under bacteriological culture conditions over the Easter weekend. It was the 35th such specimen he had placed under culture. The previous 34 had failed to grow any organisms after 48 hours and he had abandoned them. The Easter weekend meant that culture number 35 was left under incubation for 5 days. When the plate was finally examined, on 14 April 1982, it had grown a host of pure colonies of slightly curved bacteria. From then on, culture periods were all extended for 5 days – and 11 more specimens grew the new bacteria.

Bacteria had been seen in specimens of stomach material as long ago as 1874 by a Dr A. Böttcher, but he described them as spiral organisms, rather than gently curving rods, and they probably were not the same as Dr Marshall's organisms. However, by 1975 Dr H. W. Steer in Britain was describing short spiral bacteria in large numbers adhering to the stomach lining cells, and by 1979 the team in Perth was describing similar bacteria, except that they were now described as curved rather than spiral.

The bacteriologist in that team, Dr J. R. Warren, pointed out that the new bacteria were found in areas of gastritis in the stomach wall – as shown by masses of white blood cells (polymorphs), which had gathered there to deal with infection. By 1981 the team had examined many stomach ulcer biopsy specimens, and most showed the curved bacteria in great numbers and the usual signs – polymorph invasion – of gastritis. Could the newly found bacteria be the cause of the infection, of the gastritis, and of the ulcers that many of the specimens showed?

Quite by chance, one of the participants in the study had been given the antibiotic tetracycline for an infection. His ulcer symptoms disappeared, and a second biopsy showed that the gastritis had also vanished, along with the bacteria. This was the stimulus to Dr Marshall's research. He had to find some way to grow the bacterium in the laboratory, so that it could be examined in more detail. This led to the famous 'Easter culture' of 1982.

By 1985 Dr Marshall had reported in detail on 267 people with duodenal and gastric ulcers infected with the new bacterium, then called *Campylobacter*, but now called *Helicobacter pylori* and abbreviated to HP. He had, in the meantime, performed the ultimate medical experiment upon himself. He had grown *Helicobacter* in his laboratory and swallowed a large dose of it! Within days he had severe ulcer symptoms, and endoscopy showed that he had severe gastritis of the type that is associated with ulcers. He had never had stomach problems in his life before that time. Only after several days of pain, and putting himself in some danger, was he persuaded to treat himself with a cocktail of antibiotics to kill the germ. The antibiotics quickly cleared the symptoms and his stomach and duodenum healed.

How does *Helicobacter* cause ulcers? To understand that, everything about it had to be discovered – from how it comes to find a niche in such a hostile acid environment to the way it damages the digestion/protection balance in the stomach. The information about it has been expanding very rapidly: there are now around 1,000 medical publications every year about HP and its remarkable relationship with human beings – its only known host.

Who has *Helicobacter*?

HP infections around the world are closely linked with poverty and overcrowding. In the developing world, many infants are infected by HP soon after birth, and 80 to 90 per cent of people in the nations of the Global South are infected by the time they are 20 years old. The rate of infection then remains at this high level for the rest of their adult life.

In the Global North, the infection rate is less than 20 per cent in people under 30 years old. It then rises at about 1 per cent per annum, levelling out eventually so that by the age of 70 around 60 to 70 per cent of the population is infected. Within the industrialized world infection rates vary, with the lowest rates being in Denmark and the highest in Japan. The UK has relatively low rates, higher than the USA but lower than Belgium, Germany, Greece and Poland. There are differences, too, within countries. Even in developed countries, people brought up in poorer areas in overcrowded houses or institutions are more likely to be infected with HP than people who were born into wealthier households, regardless of their current economic circumstances. There is no relation between HP infection and sex, smoking, blood group or alcohol consumption. Meat eaters are at no higher risk than vegetarians, and no water sources have been implicated.

All this strongly suggests that for most people the infection occurs in childhood and is transmitted from mouth to mouth or from contaminated food to mouth. However, suggestions that poor hygiene is involved have yet to explain why there is such a high HP incidence in Japan, where there is overcrowding but good hygiene.

Helicobacter in gastritis

Even in people without ulcer symptoms, indeed with no symptoms at all, HP infection produces in the stomach an inflammatory condition called chronic superficial gastritis. This remains for as long as the *Helicobacter* survives in the stomach.

Chronic superficial gastritis has been studied for many years, long before the connection with HP was made. Scandinavian researchers found, on following up many patients with it, that in a minority it gradually changed in nature to become severe atrophic gastritis. This is a condition in which the gastric lining cells gradually die off and the secretions – acid, pepsin and mucus – are lost. The average interval from superficial gastritis to atrophic gastritis was more than 37 years!

The importance of atrophic gastritis is that it may lead to gastric cancer, and this fits with several studies (in, for example, China and Colombia) linking HP infections to stomach cancer. British figures bear this out. Dr D. J. P. Barker and colleagues showed that stomach cancer deaths in different areas of Britain between 1968 and 1978 were closely related to overcrowding 30 years before, as defined by a 1936 government survey. The overcrowding was also linked at the time with very high rates of children's infections such as bronchitis, measles and diarrhoea. It could very well be that one of those infections was HP, missed by doctors at the time because there was no way to identify the germ.

However, atrophic gastritis and cancer are not the only possible consequences of HP-induced superficial gastritis. The other is peptic ulcer. It appears that different people react differently to HP infection. Those whose gastritis goes on to atrophy, and possibly cancer, have mounted a different immune response to the bacterium from those who go on to develop ulcers.

In the gastritis-to-atrophy sequence, HP appears to block the production of acid by the parietal cells (see Chapter 2) and initiates an immune response in the stomach wall that leads to the chronic gastritis with permanent loss of acid production. Eventually the stomach cells atrophy, and the risk of conversion into cancer cells rises.

In people in whom this immune response is not stimulated, and in whom gastric atrophy is very slight or absent, then HP directly stimulates gastrin secretion, which increases acid secretion and initiates ulcer formation.

In effect, you make a choice. Once infected with HP you can mount an immune response to reduce acid levels and avoid ulcers. The price you pay is to expose yourself years later to stomach cancer. If you fail to mount the immune response, your HP infection leads to increased acid levels and ulcers!

However, even this is not the whole story. The vast majority of people who harbour HP in their stomachs do not get cancer or ulcers. They all show a mild superficial gastritis, but their condition does not progress further along either path. Most never show symptoms of ulcer or even dyspepsia and never have cause to be concerned about the germs in their stomachs. Something else must occur to provoke ulcer formation.

That something is a defect in the mucus protection against acid and pepsin. In fact, *Helicobacter* may cause several defects in the mucus layer. One is a change in the ability of the mucus to repel acid, so that the hydrochloric acid produced by the parietal cells penetrates it more easily. A second defect is that the mucus layer is thinner in HP 'carriers', so that there is less to penetrate before the acid reaches the stomach cell surface. The third defect is a subtle change in the protein structure of the mucus, so that the protein-digesting enzyme pepsin can also penetrate it. So HP not only increases the stomach's production of acid, it also promotes the destruction of the layer of mucus that protects against acid and pepsin attack. The wonder is, given the very large numbers of people infected with it, that HP does not cause much more illness than it does.

An overview of the role of HP in duodenal and gastric ulcer was given by Professors Guido Tytgat and Michael Dixon in 1993. This is still, nearly 20 years later, the most complete information on the subject so far, and it is summarized in the following paragraphs.

Helicobacter in duodenal ulcer

Of more than 250 people with duodenal ulcer in Amsterdam, every one was infected with HP (if a single person who had recently taken antibiotics is excluded). According to Professors Tytgat and Dixon, a duodenal ulcer in a person not infected with HP 'is not genuine peptic ulcer disease, and some other cause' (such as NSAIDs or small-bowel disease) 'should be sought'. However, they continue, 'only a minority of individuals har-bouring *Helicobacter* will develop duodenal ulcer, with a lifetime prevalence of 10 per cent'.

So, duodenal ulcer is a complex event. In addition to the gastritis there are other influences, such as the capacity to secrete acid and pepsin (which varies from person to person), smoking and other genetic and environmental factors. How these interact determines whether someone develops a duodenal ulcer or not. Indeed, Tytgat and Dixon continue, the actual strain of *Helicobacter* that is causing the infection may make a difference. Some strains produce toxins that damage gastric and duodenal lining cells, and others contain proteins that cause much more severe gastritis than usual. One of these proteins – 120 kDa protein – is already being used as an indi-cator that a person is heading for severe ulcer disease.

Some *Helicobacter* strains contain a gene (called *cagA*) that is also associated with severe ulcer disease. This, too, is likely to be used more and more as a predictor of severe ulcer disease.

The final proof that a bacterium causes a disease, of course, comes when its eradication from the organ concerned leads to healing and cure. Tytgat and Dixon listed 27 studies involving more than 2,000 duodenal ulcer patients, in which ulcer recurrence rates were compared between patients who continued to be infected with HP after conventional ulcer treatment and patients whose infection had been eradicated by antibiotics.

The results have been astounding. Among the patients whose stomachs remained infected, the ulcer recurrence rates ranged from 20 to 100 per cent, with most studies recording that well over half the patients had further ulcers. In the vast majority of the patients whose HP had been eradicated, the ulcers never recurred. Fourteen studies recorded no recurrences at all, and in 12 studies the recurrence rate ranged from 2 to 10 per cent. Interestingly, the highest recurrence rate among the HP-free group was recorded by Dr Marshall himself, 5 of whose 23 patients (22 per cent) had ulcer relapses. However, this compared with 38 out of 47 patients whose *Helicobacter* was not eradicated – a recurrence rate of 81 per cent.

Helicobacter in gastric ulcer

It has been known for more than 100 years that gastric ulcer occurs against a background of chronic gastritis. 'Only recently', write Tytgat and Dixon, 'has it been appreciated that *Helicobacter* infection is the cause of this gastritis.'

They suggest that the gastritis is partly caused by toxins (poisons) produced by the *Helicobacter* themselves, and partly by their release of protein-digesting enzymes that literally start to digest the stomach wall. However, other possible causes of gastric ulcer they propose include bile passing upwards from the duodenum, the use of NSAIDs, a high-salt diet and cigarette smoking.

Taking NSAIDs in particular seems to need the presence of HP to cause ulcers, according to a team of gastroenterologists and rheumatologists in Glasgow. Drs A. S. Taha, R. D. Sturrock and R. I. Russell followed 50 long-term NSAID users, 30 of whom were infected with HP. Eighteen of these 30 people (60 per cent) developed gastric erosions (areas of minor ulceration) during the study, and 12 (40 per cent) developed frank ulcers. Of the 20 not infected with HP, the corresponding numbers were 5 (25 per cent) and 3

(15 per cent). The development of ulcers was very strongly linked with the presence of HP in duodenal erosions.

Not all habits, however, are harmful: some may even protect people with HP from developing ulcers and atrophy. Chief among them, according to Tytgat and Dixon, are eating large amounts of vitamin C, vitamin E, beta-carotene and trace elements. All are substances known to counteract bacterial toxins and harmful substances, known as free radicals, which are released by inflamed tissues. This is not to say that people should swallow vitamin and mineral pills to prevent ulcers. It is far better to eat the foods that are rich in them, such as vegetables, cereals and fruits.

In the past, people with an ulcer were advised to stick to a bland diet – memories of hospital meals consisting largely of milk and steamed fish haunt many older ulcer patients. This was exactly the opposite of what was needed: such diets were virtually devoid of the vitamins and minerals needed to help heal or prevent ulcers!

As for proof that gastric ulcer is linked to HP, fewer trials have been reported than for duodenal ulcer. However, in four trials involving 375 gastric ulcer patients reported in the 1990s (the decade in which most of the HP research was completed) the relapse rates ranged from 33 to 74 per cent over 3 to 12 months in those with continuing HP infection. In three of the four trials, none of the patients in whom HP was eradicated had a further ulcer in the same time, and only 7 per cent did so in the fourth.

Professors Tytgat and Dixon come to very forthright conclusions on the relationship between HP and peptic ulcer. They postulate that in any population a small proportion of individuals are born with a larger than normal mass of parietal cells. These people develop stomach-like areas of lining in their duodenum – technically called gastric metaplasia. If they are infected by HP, the presence of this metaplasia in their duodenum allows the bacteria to be established there and cause 'duodenitis' – a condition exactly like the gastritis found in gastric ulcer. Erosion and duodenal ulcer follow.

This theory has a fundamental bearing on how ulcer disease should be treated. If it is correct – and all the latest evidence supports it – then removal of acid and pepsin will help to heal an ulcer, but will not eradicate HP. The chronic inflammation will remain, and the stomach or duodenum will be susceptible to ulcer again when the treatment is stopped and acid and pepsin attack resumes. According to Tytgat and Dixon, the only way to prevent future recurrences of ulcers in any person with duodenal or gastric ulcer is to eradicate all traces of HP. Here is what they wrote in 1993:

> Duodenal ulcer recurrence, and to a lesser extent gastric ulcer recurrence, becomes a rarity after successful *Helicobacter* eradication. Sufficient evidence has been provided to justify the recommendation to treat all patients with *Helicobacter pylori*-associated duodenal and gastric disease with anti-*Helicobacter* therapy. Eradication of *Helicobacter* equals cure of duodenal ulcer disease. Unpublished information would indicate that the beneficial effect of *Helicobacter* eradication persists as long as no reinfection occurs. The same sequence of events appears to occur for *Helicobacter*-associated gastric ulcer, but more data are required for unequivocal support for this statement.

However, *Helicobacter* alone is not the whole story. Tytgat and Dixon continue:

> Infection with *Helicobacter pylori* is undoubtedly the dominant factor in peptic ulcer. However, the other contributing factors should not be ignored, but rather one should try to identify how they interact with the organism and initiate the ulcerative process. The interplay of acid attack and mucosal defence is modulated by genetics, gender, blood group, smoking, age and various physiological considerations which include acid output. These and other considerations probably explain the discrepancy between the high frequency of *Helicobacter* infection in the population and the comparatively small proportion of individuals who develop a peptic ulcer.

Until the discovery of HP, most treatments for peptic ulcer aimed to reduce the impact of acid on the ulcer. They ease the symptoms and help to heal the ulcer, but they do not affect HP and do not heal the underlying gastritis or duodenitis. The gastric and duodenal lining cells therefore remain open to further ulcers. In the 1990s, the experts became convinced that for long-term benefit in ulcer disease, attacking HP must be part of the management. We GPs (general practitioners) have been convinced, too, by the results we have had in our patients. How we have put the advice into practice is explained in Chapter 9, on the modern management of ulcers.

Diagnosing and treating ulcers

Many people with stomach pains or indigestion have their diagnosis of ulcer made by their GP on the basis of their story and a physical examination. Treatment is started without further tests or referral to a specialist, and if the symptoms resolve and show no signs of recurrence, they may never need further investigation.

However, if symptoms persist or recur, despite what would usually be adequate treatment, then tests are indicated. What you can expect when you visit hospital for such tests is described in Chapter 4.

4

Testing for an ulcer

People who, according to their history and examination, obviously have nervous dyspepsia do not need any further investigations. As they do not have ulcers, and the treatment aims only at easing their symptoms, referring them to hospital is a waste of their time and of hospital resources. Instead, they should accept their doctor's reassurance that their symptoms do not denote serious stomach or duodenal disease, and start to tackle the cause of their underlying anxiety.

Endoscopy

However, if there is any suspicion of ulcer, or of other disease that might mimic ulcer, then you may be referred for endoscopy. Endoscopes are flexible fibre-optic tubes down which the doctor can see in perfect clarity what is going on in the oesophagus, stomach and duodenum. The endoscope can be used to take pieces (biopsies) of suspicious areas of stomach lining under direct vision.

If you are asked to have an endoscopy, be prepared to starve for at least 8 hours beforehand, so that the stomach is empty and the field of view clear. Endoscopies are usually undertaken in a special endoscopy unit separate from the operating theatre suites, and consist of a day ward and the endoscopy room itself.

In the day ward you will be asked your personal details, then, just before your endoscopy, you will be given an injection to make you sleepy but not completely unconscious. It also makes you forgetful, so that afterwards you will have only the haziest memory of what you have gone through. You will be asked to wait in the day ward for several hours after the investigation, to allow the sedation to wear off. You must not drive or work for the rest of the day, as your judgement is impaired for 24 hours or so afterwards. It is best for someone to take you to and from the centre, and to look after you for the day.

Some centres let you opt for a local anaesthetic spray in the throat, which numbs the sensation of the tube and stops you retching. This is more unpleasant but avoids the need for general sedation, so that you can return home or to work as soon as the procedure is over.

The test itself takes around 20 minutes. If a biopsy is needed, be assured that it is painless, whether you have the injection or the spray.

The endoscope is so flexible that it allows examination of every area of the oesophagus, stomach and duodenum. It can even be adapted to look into the bile duct and pancreatic duct – the two small openings from the gall bladder and pancreas into the middle of the duodenum.

To endoscope or not?

There are times when an endoscopy is unavoidable, despite the availability of other less unpleasant and inconvenient tests.

- The first is when the symptoms point definitely to peptic ulcer, and initial treatment has not helped. Some hospitals still use barium X-rays first, before endoscopy is considered. If the X-ray is negative, they go on to endoscope. If the ulcer appears on X-ray, endoscopy may not be considered necessary. However, more and more hospital departments have swung away from X-rays to go straight to endoscopy.
- The second is in people whose symptoms are so severe that an operation is being considered. Every surgeon can tell of past operations to remove part of the stomach when eventually no ulcer was found. These patients had unusual forms of nervous dyspepsia and would have been much better treated medically, without surgery.
- The third is in people with gastric ulcers, in whom malignancy cannot be excluded. Duodenal ulcers are never cancerous. The way to settle this question is to take a biopsy under endoscopy from any suspicious area of the stomach, usually in the edge of the ulcer.

- The final case is in anyone who has vomited blood (haematemesis) or has passed blood in black stools (melaena). The endoscopy will identify the site of bleeding, and can be used to stop it.

X-rays

Because of the comprehensive view of the 'target area' provided by endoscopy, it has largely replaced X-rays such as barium meals as the main method of investigation of people suspected of having an ulcer.

However, barium examination still has its uses. A very small number of people, for example, are deemed unfit for endoscopy – although endoscopy is now so well established that this number is vanishingly small. In some people who have had problems with previous attempts at endoscopy, X-rays are used as the next best test.

The principle of a barium meal is simple. The X-rays cannot penetrate barium, so that it appears as a white shadow against the black background of the abdomen. It sticks to the oesophageal, stomach and duodenal lining, so that any ulcer has to be shown up as a change from the normal in their outlines. An ulcer, for example, can show as a 'punched out' or 'filled in' area on the side of the stomach or as a constant narrowing in the duodenum due to scarring.

X-rays are less accurate than endoscopy in diagnosing ulcer, as they can miss an ulcer if it is not shown in profile or even suggest an ulcer where in fact there is scarring from an old healed ulcer that is no longer causing problems. By seeing the ulcer direct, these errors should not be made by endoscopy. Some clinics use both barium X-rays and endoscopy to provide as complete a picture as possible.

If you are asked to attend for barium X-ray, just as with endoscopy you must starve for at least 8 hours beforehand to empty your stomach. You will go straight to the X-ray department, where you will be asked to drink a thick, creamy, white liquid. Your radiologist (a doctor specializing in interpreting X-rays) will watch on the screen as the liquid passes down the oesophagus, into the stomach, then through into the duodenum.

You may also be asked to swallow a fizzy drink, or the barium may have 'fizz' in it. This distends the stomach, giving the radiologist a better view of the contrast between the stomach lining and the barium. You may be strapped to a table and turned in several directions – even almost upside down – to give a view into every nook and cranny. Every few minutes the radiologist will stop and take photographs, so that he or she can later identify suspicious appearances on the television monitor screen.

Like endoscopy, barium X-rays take around 20 minutes, but they may drag on longer if some appearance demands extra attention, so be prepared to spend several hours in the X-ray department. X-rays are not as uncomfortable as endoscopy, but you should be warned that you can become constipated afterwards, as the barium can pack fairly solidly into the large bowel and rectum. So make sure that you open your bowels regularly for the next few days. You may even have to take advice from your GP or radiologist about how to cope with it. Eating plenty of fruit and drinking copious amounts of water is usually enough. A mild stool softener can also help, for example lactulose, two tablespoonsful each evening.

Testing for *Helicobacter pylori*

Endoscopy

A big advantage of endoscopy is that it allows the gastroenterologist to take away a piece of the suspected ulcer tissue, or of what looks like gastritis, for examination. This allows direct identification of HP under the microscope. Only a decade or so after Dr Marshall's original work, every hospital laboratory had the ability to see HP in stomach or duodenal biopsy specimens. All that is needed is the correct staining technique, and the curved bacteria with their hair-like flagellae can be clearly identified.

Cultures

The material from the stomach can also be cultured under the correct conditions to grow colonies of *Helicobacter*. This offers the chance to test the colonies against the killing power of different antibiotics, the most effective of which can then be used in treatment.

There may even be no need to pass an endoscope down the throat to obtain specimens of *Helicobacter*. Dr E. Perez-Trallero and colleagues, of San Sebastian, Spain, recommend their 'capsule on a string' method. Instead of using an endoscope, they tie an absorbent string to an ordinary capsule, similar to any capsule containing a drug to be swallowed. However, the capsule contains nothing! It is just a way to get the string down into the stomach.

After around an hour, the string is pulled up again – minus the now dissolved capsule – with no discomfort. It is placed on a bacterial culture plate, which will grow any *Helicobacter* that stuck to the string while it was in the stomach! The Spanish team claim that it is much more user-friendly than endoscopy, and just as accurate in confirming that the HP is present.

Urea breath test

It may not be necessary to identify *Helicobacter* at all to show that it is present in the stomach. HP possesses a powerful enzyme, urease, which breaks down the waste substance urea that is present in all human tissues. If you swallow a small amount of urea 'labelled' with a tiny amount of radioactive carbon, and your stomach contains active *Helicobacter*, the urea will be broken down much faster than normal, and the radioactive carbon will appear faster and in higher amounts than normal in the breath.

This discovery has led to the development of the urea breath test, in which you will be asked to swallow a tasteless fluid, then give samples of your breath. The amount of radioactivity in the sample not only confirms that you are infected with HP, but may even indicate the extent of the infection.

The breath test is particularly useful where it is difficult to get culture material, or where the infection is only slight. Its main use may prove to be in follow-up, to check for continuing infection or reinfection in people who have been given treatment to eradicate HP. It is also, of course, much more user-friendly than endoscopy or even the capsule on a string. There is no need to worry about the dose of radioactivity used. It is tiny, and is quickly gone from the body, so it poses no health risk in itself.

When the breath test was being developed, samples of breath were taken for 2 hours after swallowing the drink, which is simply a 50 ml glass of water into which a small gelatine capsule of urea has been dissolved. Now most hospitals accept that all that is needed is a breath sample taken 40 minutes after drinking. You will be asked to exhale gently through a disposable plastic straw into a test tube.

Blood tests

Finally, there are blood tests to detect antibodies to HP. The body's response to any infection is to produce antibodies in an attempt to fight off the bacterium causing it. Antibodies are unique to the particular bacterial strain causing the infection, so the finding of antibodies against HP in your blood means that you must have been infected by it in the past. As most untreated HP infections are lifelong, such a finding almost certainly means that you are still infected.

The current blood test, technically called an enzyme-linked immunosorbent assay (ELISA), is simple, reliable and relatively cheap. ELISA tests are used to detect the proportion of people in a population infected by HP and perhaps to screen possible ulcer patients before endoscopy. A negative result points against a duodenal ulcer; a positive one may lead doctors to go ahead with endoscopy. Most doctors would caution against deciding that an ulcer is present on a positive blood test alone.

Current family practice in 2011: almost instant diagnosis

One enormously important advance in testing for HP is the on-the-spot breath test available now to all GPs in Britain for use in the surgery. It has been so successful that the doctors in the practices with which I have been privileged to be associated use it routinely in all people whom they think could be infected. All you are asked to do is to swallow a tablet, powder or soluble tablet, and then breathe out through a straw into a container. The breath sample may be analysed in the surgery or sent to the local laboratory, where the results are almost instantly available. A positive test means that the treatment can start, and other investigations can be shelved or postponed. If the symptoms disappear, there is no need for further tests. It has been a huge boon for doctors and patients alike, and a huge saving in time, expertise and costs.

5

When it is not an ulcer

It must be obvious after reading the section on nervous dyspepsia that pain in the pit of the stomach is not always due to ulcers. However, dyspepsia is not the only problem that mimics ulcer: there are others that need urgent investigation and treatment, and it is best to know something about them. That is because, of all the mistakes that people make in trying to diagnose their own medical conditions, the most common is to assume that pain high in the stomach is due to an ulcer or indigestion. They then self-treat with an antacid – and this can be a serious, and sometimes fatal, mistake.

I can best illustrate this with a few case histories.

The 'missed' coronary

James, aged 57, complained of indigestion to his wife one evening after a heavy meal and a drink or two. The pain was a dull ache right in what he described as 'the centre of the upper stomach', below the breastbone, between the ribs. He swallowed an antacid, went to bed and took around an hour to get to sleep after tossing around for a while with the pain. Around 3.00 a.m. he woke. This time his pain, still in the same place, was much worse and the antacid did not help. His wife became worried because he was cold and clammy, and sweating profusely. She called the doctor, who recognized the symptoms and signs of a heart attack (a coronary thrombosis). He was given injections to kill the pain and undo the clotting process in his heart, and admitted to hospital.

As he began to recover, James admitted to his doctor that he had been having this dull aching pain quite often in the previous few weeks. It had come on after meals, which was why he had assumed it was indigestion or an ulcer. Being a busy man, much stressed at work, he had not taken the time off to see his doctor, and had treated himself with antacids bought from the local pharmacy. Although they had not helped immediately, the pain had always subsided when he rested. Asked if he had noticed the pain on exercise, such as walking or climbing stairs, he replied that he hardly ever exercised. He lived and worked in a single-storey building, and always used a lift when visiting business colleagues! He had noticed the pain occasionally when driving, but he had assumed that this was pressure from his seat belt on an irritated stomach.

Assuming pain in the upper stomach, or even in the lower chest, is indigestion is the most common mistake of all. Heart pain, or angina, is not always in the chest or left-sided (though it is very rarely right-sided). It can be central, and confined to the upper abdomen.

It can be difficult to differentiate between the qualities of ulcer pain and heart pain. Both can be described as dull and aching, or boring and gnawing. However, neither is likely to be burning or sharp. Tightness or a gripping sensation that prevents deep breathing points towards angina, rather than ulcer.

It can also be difficult to distinguish between them on timing – heart and stomach pains can both be brought on by a heavy meal or by excess alcohol. However, stomach or duodenal ulcer pain is rarely induced by exercise, and does not disappear on rest – fundamental properties of angina. James missed his own diagnosis partly because he never exercised! The clue lay in the lack of relief from antacids, and the occasional spike of pain when driving, when his blood pressure and heart rate may have been pushed up by stress, and his narrowed coronary arteries became unable, temporarily, to cope.

The 'missed' gallstones

William, a slim, fit 65-year-old, had his first bout of pain one evening while sitting with his feet up at home. It started about half an hour after his evening meal. It, like James' pain, was in the pit of his stomach, if anything slightly to the right of centre. It hit him suddenly and persisted for around 3 hours before stopping, just as suddenly. It came in waves, worsening for around 10 minutes at a time, then dying off, though not completely, until the next bout.

William described it as a severe stomach cramp, coming in spasms, and at its height very severe, making him 'want to curl up'. However, once the bout was over he felt well, though he was apprehensive about it returning.

William, like James, blamed the pain on indigestion. The meal he had eaten before it started was not unusual for him: it was pasta, followed by cheese and biscuits. Also like James, he took an antacid preparation and rested until the pain was over. He assumed, from what he read in his home medicine encyclopaedia and had gathered from the internet, that this must be acute indigestion and decided to avoid cheese in the future!

However, avoiding cheese did not help. He called the doctor when he suffered a repeat bout of the same pain a few days later. It came on at around the same time and lasted just as long. This time he had eaten fish shallow-fried in oil and a baked potato – being health minded, he had for years avoided fats. What worried him about this bout was that the pain was now passing through to his back, around his right shoulder blade, and he was being sick with it.

His doctor found that he was quite tender to the right side of the upper abdomen, just under the rib margin. He was given an injection of a painkiller and an antispasmodic to ease the spasm, and was referred for X-rays. They showed what the doctor suspected – a cluster of small gallstones lying in his gall bladder.

William was astonished. He had read that people with gallstones were 'fat, fair, fertile, forty and female', and he was certainly none of them! His doctor explained that this stereotype was well wide of the truth. Many men have gallstones, they are not necessarily fat, nor is it necessary for them to have a high-fat diet, and fair-haired people are no more likely to grow stones than dark-haired ones. In fact, the highest incidence of gallstones in the world is in indigenous North American people.

The clues to the cause of his pain lay in the sudden onset, the cramp-like character, the bias towards the right side, and the fact that it also bored towards his right shoulder blade. The second bout, with the complication of vomiting, pointed strongly to the possession of several gallstones, passing one by one from gall bladder into the bowel through the bile duct.

William's pain was cured by surgery to remove the gall bladder and the stones within it. He turned out to have very high blood cholesterol levels: he was given drugs to lower them and to keep them low for the foreseeable future.

The 'missed' pancreatitis

Henry's pain was in the pit of his stomach. Unlike the others, though, it was a fairly constant, persistent ache for most of his waking hours. Fifty years old, he had had it for a few years and put it down largely to indigestion caused by his irregular eating habits. He found the best way to relieve it was a little alcohol. In fact, he was willing to admit that he found alcohol a good way to relieve most of his problems. He drank well over the recommended upper limit of 21 standard drinks a week, without ever getting outrageously drunk.

What brought him to his doctor was the fact that he was now passing bulky, foul-smelling, pale stools. He still had a voracious appetite but he was losing weight. Recently, the pain had started to 'bore into' his back, so that he felt it in the middle of his spine, as well as in his abdomen. He had heard that this might be a sign of a perforating ulcer, and he was beginning to panic.

This combination of symptoms led his doctor to do a series of blood tests that proved he had an inflamed pancreas – or chronic relapsing pancreatitis. This is a condition closely linked with excess alcohol consumption. The bulky stools were due to poor fat digestion, because the pancreas was now failing. The blood tests also showed some liver damage.

If Henry wants to survive he must stop drinking. He has been told, but whether he can do so remains to be seen. It is up to him.

The 'missed' irritable bowel

Robert, aged 27, was a nervous young man, very insecure in his job and his social relationships. His main complaint was of discomfort in the pit of the stomach, along with a bloated feeling shortly after eating any meal.

The discomfort was hardly a pain, but it was so regular that Robert thought that it must be an ulcer or 'something similar'. He was very anxious to find the cause and have it treated. Only when he started to expand on all of his complaints did his doctor get the whole picture and reach the correct diagnosis.

Robert was also experiencing pain in his lower abdomen, mainly on the left side. It was relieved sometimes, but not always, by opening his bowels, and when he did so he passed a shower of rabbity, pellet-like hard stools. Sometimes the stools were ribbon-shaped or pencil-like, and he often felt the urge to do still more after rising from the toilet.

The history alone, and the lack of anything to show physical disease, was enough to persuade his doctor that Robert had irritable bowel syndrome. However, he needed considerable persuasion that he did not need extensive investigations to rule out serious disease such as ulcers or cancer. He is now being treated with antispasmodic drugs to relieve cramps in the bowel, and is receiving psychological support for his anxiety state.

The 'missed' stomach cancer

John, at 52, had had mild dyspepsia for around 20 years, which he had controlled well by himself with chewy antacid tablets he bought from the local pharmacy. He was so used to it that he never consulted his doctor about it. However, for a few weeks he had been feeling different. He had begun to feel discomfort in the pit of his stomach – more of a vague unease than a pain. It was linked to the inability to finish a large meal and a sense of fullness in his stomach after a much smaller meal than normal.

For a while he assumed that this was just a different sort of dyspepsia, and tried to treat it himself with cimetidine, at that time a new acid-suppressing drug recently released for sale over the pharmacy counter. He gave it a week's trial, but felt no better. Discussing his symptoms with the pharmacist, he was advised to see his doctor, which he reluctantly did, believing he was wasting her time.

She listened to his story, and to the additional facts that his appetite was not as good as it was and that he had recently lost half a stone (3 kg) in weight. She heard the alarm bells ringing and examined his abdomen. She could feel a vague mass, not much more than a difference in resistance to her fingers, about halfway between the navel and the breastbone.

Sent immediately for further tests, John was found to have a stomach cancer, which was operated on within the week. At operation there were no signs of spread beyond his stomach, so there are hopes that he will survive in good health for many years to come.

John's case is a vital lesson for anyone with vague abdominal troubles. Anyone who notices any new digestive symptom in middle age should quickly seek medical advice. It is crucial that cancers are diagnosed as early as possible, and that will only happen if even trivial new symptoms are brought to your doctor's notice early.

The cardinal symptoms of gastric cancer are not necessarily pain at first, but include vague discomfort, changes in feelings about food, loss of appetite and loss of weight. Stomach cancers are particularly common in Finland, Japan, Chile and Iceland, perhaps because of a combination of eating habits and heredity. In Britain, stomach cancers are more common than normal in people with blood group A (as opposed to the prevalence of blood group O in ulcer cases), in people with pernicious anaemia and in people who have had previous ulcer surgery. About 1 in 5 people who develop stomach cancer give a history of many years of indigestion.

However, do not be frightened by these figures. Stomach cancers are becoming rapidly much rarer than they were in Britain and the rest of the developed world. This may be linked to better food storage, so that we consume fewer nitrates, chemicals known to be associated with cancerous changes in the stomach. Initial fears that long-term treatment with drugs such as omeprazole, which completely suppress stomach acid production, may also stimulate cancer have been allayed. This will be described in more detail in the chapter on drug treatment.

In Japan, the problem of gastric cancer was perceived as so great that a mass endoscopy screening for it was started. It has already shown benefits, in that early cancers have been detected that are clearly curable with surgery. The British stomach cancer figures are so low that the expense of healthy population screening would be much too high for the potential benefit. However, people with cases of stomach cancer or pernicious anaemia in their family may well benefit from screening programmes in the future.

I have used male case histories to illustrate the pitfalls of assuming that pain in the upper abdomen is necessarily to do with the stomach or duodenum. This is to emphasize that men are just as prone to abdominal disorders as women – contrary to popular beliefs promoted by older home medicine encyclopaedias, some current women's magazines and more recently, sadly, the internet. However, each case history could apply equally to women. The symptoms are just the same in the two sexes.

6

Managing your health: food, fitness and stress

Now that your diagnosis has been made, and you have to live with your ulcer, can you help yourself by altering your eating habits and lifestyle?

Eating correctly

Naturally, the first question that everyone with an ulcer asks is about diet: 'Can I heal my ulcer on diet alone, or at least with diet and antacids?'

If, by diet, you mean special foods and a special way of cooking, then the answer is a decisive *no*. For many years, doctors misguidedly recommended bland diets for people with an ulcer. Steamed fish, milk puddings, mashed potatoes, and what appeared to be strict avoidance of any food that had any taste or bite to it, was the order of the day.

Frankly, those diets were disastrous. People hated them, and all enjoyment of food was ruined. Their lives, and often the lives of their closest family, were made miserable by the tyranny and the dullness of the 'ulcer kitchen'. They were also unhealthy diets, as many of the vitamins were boiled or steamed out of them. Taken to extremes, the combination of milk and antacids led in the past to 'milk–alkali syndrome', in which calcium levels in the blood rose so steeply that stones formed in the kidneys, leading to kidney failure.

We now know that if you have an ulcer you need to eat as varied a combination of foods as possible. That means meats, fish, cereals, vegetables and fruit. If a particular food repeatedly upsets you, then avoid it – but this should be unnecessary, as very few true ulcer patients react badly to a single food or group of foods. As mentioned in Chapter 1, food allergy is very rare, and not connected to ulcer disease.

Some people with an ulcer do feel uncomfortable after fatty meals. If this is your experience, cut out fried foods – grill instead – and trim the fat from your meat. However, intolerance to fat is more likely to be a sign of gall bladder trouble than of peptic ulcer, so tell your doctor about it.

Do eat foods likely to help to heal ulcers, such as those rich in vitamins C and E. That means fruit, cereals and green vegetables lightly cooked (preferably steamed or stir-fried in vegetable oil) and not boiled for ages in water.

More important than any of the above advice on food, however, is *not to go hungry*. Organize your eating so that you have three or four regular meals a day, at regular intervals. Many of those with an ulcer rush down a cup of coffee for breakfast, have a sandwich for lunch, and leave their main meal for the evening. They snack occasionally between meals, often to ease the odd niggle in their stomach.

This is exactly the wrong way to eat. You must start the day with a good breakfast, even if it means rising an hour earlier to prepare it. That extra hour is worth it! For breakfast, tea, fruit juice, toast, porridge or cereal, a scrambled egg, a kipper, or even grilled lean bacon and egg, is the perfect start to an antiulcer day. It neutralizes the early morning acid production and sets you up with your energy store for the day. A small sandwich with your mid-morning break will keep the morning acid/pepsin attack at bay.

Lunch could be soup and a sandwich or a pasta dish, followed by fruit. Then comes a small snack around 4.00 p.m., and dinner at 6.30 or 7.00 p.m. Dinner need not be a massive affair. A tasty starter and a reasonable main course of meat, poultry or fish with a variety of vegetables should satisfy you and keep down the evening surplus of acid. If you are often wakened at night, then a small glass of milk just before sleeping can put it off.

Keeping fit

This sounds a very fattening programme of eating, but it is not, provided you keep fit and active with exercise. That can be anything from a regular brisk walk to running, cycling, dancing, aerobics, swimming, training or a fitness programme at the gym. If you had a sport, such as football or hockey, think of taking it up again. In most sports centres there are 'old crocks' indoors five-a-side teams ready to take on anyone! The aim is to get breathless three times a week. This will control your weight and help your fitness. It will also make you feel good about yourself, perhaps for the first time in years.

There is no evidence that keeping fit will help heal ulcers, but it will prevent you putting on the excess weight that many ulcer patients put on while eating to ease their pain. It will also help to disabuse you of the idea that may have crept into your mind that you are somehow an invalid. People with an ulcer are not in general invalids, physically or mentally. They have one health problem – a breakdown in the acid/pepsin:mucus protection balance in the stomach. In every other way they should be healthy, and able to take exercise like anyone else. So go to it!

Exercises that you should avoid, however, especially if you have heartburn, include bending over, lifting heavy weights, and 'explosive' field athletic events, such as throwing the discus, hammer and javelin. Golf, for example, is a better regular exercise than bowls or gardening, if these involve constant bending down or digging.

Lying flat can also stimulate heartburn, so that sleeping on three or more pillows or putting 9-inch (23 cm) blocks under the head of the bed can help keep the acid where it belongs, below the diaphragm. It will help, too, if you avoid tight clothing around the waist.

Bed-rest

Only a few years ago the only treatment thought to help ulcers to heal was a combination of bed-rest, constant antacid treatment and stopping smoking. Smoking deserves a chapter on its own, which comes next, but bed-rest and antacids are now known not to have any influence on the long-term course of ulcer disease. Resting in bed to 'allow an ulcer to heal' seems reasonable advice, and stomach ulcer size, as shown on X-ray, certainly diminishes while its owner rests; but as soon as he or she is upright again it is very likely to recur. It may certainly make the sufferer feel more comfortable, but it is no long-term answer or cure.

Tackling stress

Stress is popularly claimed as a cause of ulcers. Duodenal ulcers are looked upon as the 'businessman's disease', in that they are seen as the penalty of the pressures of modern life. It seems unlikely, however, that our worries today are greater than the worries of previous generations, who were apparently remarkably free of ulcers.

We do know for certain, however, that emotions have a huge influence on our stomach and duodenum. As long ago as 1833 Dr W. Beaumont, a Canadian physician, published his observations on the stomach of his patient Alexis St Martin. St Martin had been shot in the abdomen, and survived with a fistula – an opening between the stomach and the abdominal skin – through which Dr Beaumont could look directly at the inside of the stomach.

He found that the stomach wall changed colour and glistened with secretions almost instantaneously with changes in St Martin's emotions – such as anger, hunger and pleasure. The colour change was due to changes in the blood supply to the lining cells, stimulating the secretion of the gastric juices. However, the obvious changes in the stomach did not correlate at all with any symptoms. St Martin did not complain of ulcer-type pain or indigestion, even when his stomach wall was blushing furiously and producing litres of juice. Presumably his mucus defence system was more than enough to cope with the extra acid attack.

The experiment was repeated more than 100 years later, by Drs S. Wolf and H. G. Wolff, in 1947. Their subject, Tom, like St Martin, had a gastric fistula. In Tom, hostility and resentment caused obvious congestion of the stomach lining, which easily bled.

St Martin and Tom apart, there is little hard evidence to show that worry and stress cause ulcers. However, they may well make already established ulcers worse. An 'ulcer personality' that predisposes to ulcers probably does not exist, but if you already have an ulcer it is important to learn to react to stresses without becoming angry or over-anxious.

How do you do that? One of the most useless pieces of advice ever given – and it is given so often – is to 'take it easy and relax'. It does not explain how to follow that advice, so it worries you more, and makes you less relaxed. And most people who are worried and under stress are like that because they see no way around their problems. You must solve your problems *before* you can relax.

One way to start coping better is to make an objective review of your own personality and lifestyle, your worries and fears, and how you react to them. This may be the first time you have faced them coolly and logically. If so, that in itself may show that you have hidden some truths about yourself from yourself.

The purpose of your review is not to learn how to avoid meeting stress, for example by leaving your job for an easier one, but to learn how to react better to the stresses you meet in your present environment. You will enjoy meeting the challenges in life more if you can cope with stress without pouring acid and pepsin into your stomach each time you meet with it!

You know if you are reacting badly to stress if you have the following symptoms apart from your peptic ulcer pain:

- a tension headache like a vice over the surface of the skull, from the muscles at the back of the neck to the ones behind your eyebrows;
- insomnia;
- palpitations;
- bouts of diarrhoea alternating with constipation;
- loss of appetite.

Whether the stress is related to anxieties at work or home, ask yourself the following:

- Am I coping with my everyday responsibilities?
- If not, how can I change my life so that I can?
- Who can I ask to help me change in the right direction?
- Am I suppressing feelings of anger, fear or worry that I should have openly expressed to the person who can do something about them, or at least help me share them?
- Am I neglecting an important area of my life by devoting too much time to another?

- If so, how can I take practical steps to change that?
- Do I relax enough, at any time of day, and forget my worries?
- If not, when can I spare the time to do so and what should I do?

The answers to all these questions need action from you, and not your doctor, or even your family or work colleagues. You must take the first step to a better approach to stress: you are on your own until you have done so. From then on, others can help.

Now, suppose that you have taken the right decisions:

- Your excessive workload is being shared with a new colleague or assistant.
- You have delegated that next trip abroad to your deputy to spend more time with your family.
- Your bank manager is now helping you over that financial worry that has cost you your sleep for weeks.
- You have finally had that long-needed parental chat with your teenage daughter, and found it not so bad after all.

Yet you are still tense and anxious, for no reason! What can you do about it? First, accept you are not alone. A survey of American families showed that only 18 per cent of them felt that they had no need to reduce the stress in their lives!

Second, you can try one of the relaxation techniques described below. Choose the one that appeals most to you and stick with it for a while. It should be of help, and could go some way towards controlling your gastric acid output – and any ulcer symptoms.

Progressive muscle relaxation

This is the simplest technique. It is used to ease phobias and help bring down high blood pressure, which if the stomachs of St Martin and Tom are anything to go by, should also reduce stomach secretions. Lie down in a quiet room and systematically tense and relax the different groups of muscles in your body, concentrating on each in turn until you have covered them all. Start and finish where you like: I prefer to start with the eyelids, scalp, neck and shoulders, then to progress to the arms, wrists and fingers, the back, chest muscles, stomach and hips, before finishing with the thighs, calves, feet and toes. If you need more detail, it is in *You Must Relax*, by E. Jacobson, published by McGraw-Hill, New York (1978).

Meditation

The practice of meditation to induce relaxation stems from the East, largely from yoga and transcendental meditation (TM).

Yoga relaxation exercises concentrate on taking up particular physical postures and controlling breathing. TM involves taking part in twice-daily sessions, sitting in a comfortable upright position, breathing slowly and peacefully, and repeating a special phrase or mantra.

Both are fairly simple relaxation techniques, but some teachers complicate their use with mystical and philosophical ideas from Eastern religions, which can be off-putting. However, the relaxing effect of the exercises does not depend at all on acceptance of the teacher's religious views, so if you find they work, go ahead without embarrassment! Many evening classes offer yoga without the religious extras, so you can try it for yourself without the fear of proselytization!

If you find yoga too much, try t'ai chi or qigong, two methods of exercising originating in China, in which groups of people go through a series of slow exercises designed to improve their balance. They are great fun, as well as relaxing: the local qigong group (of about 20 60-somethings) in our rural area has markedly improved their wellbeing, including that of the three or four with digestive disturbances.

The relaxation response

An American doctor, Herbert Benson, adapted TM to suit a more Western audience; he calls it the 'relaxation response'. The following points outline the system briefly, which should be practised twice a day.

- Sit quietly and comfortably.
- Close your eyes.
- Relax all your muscles, as in progressive muscle relaxation.
- Breathe rhythmically through your nose. Be aware of your breathing. As you breathe out, say the word 'one' silently.
- Continue for 20 minutes. Then complete the session by sitting quietly for a few minutes.

Do not worry about whether you are successful at achieving a deep level of relaxation. Keep passive, and allow relaxation to occur at its own pace. When distracting thoughts occur, ignore them and keep repeating the word 'one'.

The Alexander technique

This system of relaxation exercises was devised by an Australian actor, E. M. Alexander, at the end of the nineteenth century. His exercises are still relevant today.

He believed that we perform wrongly many of our everyday actions, such as sitting and walking. This puts strain on our bodies, and affects the way we breathe. We tend to slump in on ourselves, bending our backs and compressing our ribs inwards, limiting the amount of air we breathe in and causing the spinal muscles to stiffen. The result is bad posture and muscle pains, which lead to physical and mental stresses.

The Alexander technique helps people to breathe and relax more naturally. It is taught individually by qualified Alexander instructors, who study for three years at an approved training school. Sessions take from 45 minutes to 1 hour, and instructors can come to your home. Most people find three to four lessons are enough to learn the techniques that particularly help them, and continue to practise on their own.

My own favourite Alexander exercise is so relaxing that it can send you to sleep. All you need to do is to lie flat on the floor, on your back, with a book under the back of your head of precisely the right thickness to keep your head straight on the neck, with chin neither bent down towards your chest or tilted upwards towards the ceiling.

Once you are settled in this position, relax all your muscles, from toes to scalp, so that you are perfectly comfortable. You will be amazed how easy that is, even on a hard floor. Stay like that for at least 5 minutes, then stretch the whole of your right side downwards, as far as your arm, torso, leg and foot will go, leaving your head behind on the book and your left side as it was. Stretch for 15 to 20 seconds and then relax again. Do that five or six times, then relax completely for half a minute. Then do the same with the left side, leaving the right side as it was. Repeat the exercise around five to six times on both sides, then relax in the same position for

10 minutes. You may well find that you snooze off for a while: if you do, that is good. Do this two or three times a day, when you can, and you will find it addictive – but it is a much healthier addiction than any drug!

If you would like to know more, contact the Society of Teachers of the Alexander Technique (see Useful addresses). Your local physiotherapist, as well as giving advice about relaxation, will usually have the address of your nearest local Alexander teacher. She may even *be* your nearest Alexander teacher, as many physiotherapists have this skill as the second string to their bow.

Drinking and smoking

Like stress, drinking and smoking do not appear to initiate ulcers, but they can make an ulcer worse once it is established and active.

Spirits do irritate the stomach (alcohol stimulates acid secretion), and can cause ulcer pain and bleeding, even when diluted half-and-half with water. People with ulcer symptoms should therefore avoid alcohol, except with food, and probably at no stronger concentration than a glass of wine or beer. There is no need to do without alcohol completely, unless you have an alcohol problem.

Smoking is a different matter. If you continue to smoke cigarettes while you have an ulcer, it will not heal. This is true even if you are given drugs proven to heal ulcers, such as the H_2 antagonists cimetidine and ranitidine. So it is vital to stop smoking. How you can do so is in the next chapter.

7

Stopping smoking

If you have ulcers and smoke, then the most charitable judgement is that you have not yet heard or read the facts. Which means that you must have been living somewhere other than the surface of this planet! However, being charitable, you have the benefit of my doubt. Read on, and if by the end of this chapter you are not a confirmed non-smoker, then throw the book away. Because nothing else you read will be of any help to you. No amount of medical or surgical treatment will prevent you from continuing to have your ulcers – and a host of other unpleasant illnesses besides.

No one who takes heed of the modern media can fail to have heard that smoking causes heart attacks, chronic bronchitis, lung cancer and damage to the circulation in the limbs. The message that it also causes cancer of the bladder and kidney, and is a powerful promoter of stomach and duodenal ulcers, is probably less well known – but these are facts too, and not scaremongering. If you continue to smoke, your risks of all these diseases rise: just because you have an ulcer does not mean that you cannot develop all these other diseases, too.

So, if you are having a struggle giving up or have not yet been persuaded of the need to give up, please read the rest of this chapter. Non-smokers can self-righteously skip it!

The effects of smoking

Virtually all adult smokers started their habit as teenagers, when they were too immature to think of its long-term consequences. If you are still a non-smoker by the age of 20, it is odds on that you will remain so for the rest of your life. By this time you have learned sense!

Your first cigarette made you nauseous, dizzy and ill as the poisons in the smoke entered your brain. New smokers have to

be persuaded by their friends to continue. Despite the highly publicized 1994 denials to the US Congressional Committee by the
American tobacco barons that tobacco is not addictive, this pattern
of behaviour – of wishing to switch your peers on to your own
habit – is a classic sign of addiction.

Within days the nicotine addiction takes hold. Soon the smoker
feels unwell without a cigarette. The withdrawal symptoms have
started – another classic sign of addiction. From then on it is down-
hill all the way. Few smokers can manage to stop at one or two
cigarettes a day: within a year or so, most are smoking 20 or more,
and many are smoking 60. This gradual increase in the dose needed
to feed the habit is the third classic sign of addiction.

To doctors like myself, who have had to comfort so many families
in which smoking has directly led to the deaths of loved ones only
in their forties and fifties, it is frankly incredible that anyone should
wish to light up a single cigarette. But to a smoker, the addiction is
more important than life itself! This is particularly true of a smoker
with an ulcer, because cigarettes directly prevent healing of ulcers –
and that means raising the risks of bleeding and perforation. Both
of these complications, described in Chapter 2, have caused many
early deaths in otherwise completely healthy people.

How does smoking make ulcers worse? Its direct effects are caused
by nicotine and carbon monoxide. If you smoke only one cigarette
a day you have enough of each in your bloodstream to reduce the
chance of your ulcer healing.

Nicotine is a powerful vasoconstrictor: that is, it narrows disas-
trously the small arteries that supply the stomach and duodenal
lining cells with oxygen and nutrients. This damages the ability to
make the protective mucus, but at the same time it stimulates the
secretion of acid and pepsin. It therefore pushes the acid/pepsin:
mucus protection equation in exactly the wrong way.

If that were not bad enough, the carbon monoxide reduces
the oxygen content of the blood, so that the blood that does
pass through the narrowed vessels is carrying less oxygen than
it should. This combination of low blood flow and even lower
oxygen content, plus the direct effect of the poisonous carbon
monoxide on the cells themselves, has a disastrous effect on the
cells in the stomach and duodenal linings.

Ulcer healing is critically dependent on the oxygen supply, and even the slightest carbon monoxide content delays healing. If it is high, as it is in a smoker of 20 cigarettes or more per day, healing becomes impossible. There will always be an open sore in the stomach or duodenum, with all the potential that has for catastrophic bleeding or perforation. Even at the lowest levels of carbon monoxide and nicotine, as measured in non-smokers who passively smoke other people's cigarettes, healing must be delayed.

Add to that the effects your smoking has on your other vital organs – in particular the lungs and heart – and the motivation to stop is very strong. So here is the motivation put into words!

Consider the following facts about smoking:

- Smoking plays a main part in most deaths from heart disease, chronic lung disease (such as chronic bronchitis and emphysema), and lung cancer.
- Smokers are more than twice as likely to have a fatal heart attack as non-smokers, and the risk rises with each added cigarette per day.
- Men under 45 years old who smoke 25 or more cigarettes per day have a 10 to 15 times greater chance of a fatal heart attack than non-smokers.
- In developed countries one-third of men die before they reach 65: most of these deaths are the direct result of smoking, the main 'widow-maker'.
- Forty per cent of all heavy smokers die before their 65th birthday; of the others, many are disabled by angina, bronchitis, heart failure or the need for leg amputations, all of which are due to smoking.
- Only 10 per cent of smokers survive to 75 years in good health: most non-smokers are healthy at that age.
- Forty per cent of all deaths due to cancer in Britain are caused by lung cancer: only 7 of 441 male British doctors who died of lung cancer had never smoked.
- Only 1 in 60 non-smokers develops lung cancer (even then they may have been passive smokers): the corresponding figure for heavy smokers is 1 in 6.
- Other smoking-related cancers include tumours of the tongue,

throat, larynx, pancreas, kidney, bladder and cervix: one-third of all cancers are caused directly by smoking.

Excuses, excuses

Have I persuaded you to stop yet? Yes? Good. No? Is your argument one of the dozens of excuses doctors hear every day to support the need to carry on? Here they are, with my responses.

My uncle/father/grandfather smoked 20 a day and lived to 75. We all know someone like that, but we forget all the others who died long before their time. The long odds-on chances are that you will be one of the many, and not one of the few.

People who don't smoke also have lung disease. True, but more than 98 per cent of all people with serious chronic lung disease are smokers or ex-smokers, and for the few whose disease is inherited, smoking makes it much worse.

People who don't smoke also have peptic ulcer. Also true, but when they are treated with ulcer-healing drugs, their ulcers heal. Ulcers in people who continue to smoke do not heal, or take much longer to do so.

Moderation in everything is my rule: I'm only a moderate smoker. Do you accept moderation in lead or arsenic poisoning, dangerous driving or violence? There is no safe lower limit to nicotine or carbon monoxide poisoning, so the idea of moderate smoking is nonsense.

I can cut down, rather than stop. You can, but it will not help. People who cut down usually take more puffs from each cigarette, leave a smaller butt, and end up with the same amount of nicotine and carbon monoxide in their bloodstream and mucosal cells. The only answer is to stop completely.

I'm just as likely to be run over in the road as to die from smoking. In Britain, traffic causes 15 deaths a day. Chronic bronchitis due to smoking causes 100, as do lung cancer and heart attacks, which is 20 times as many daily deaths. Of every 1,000 young men who smoke, on average one will be murdered, six will die on the roads, and 250 will die prematurely because they smoke. Among them will be around 15 who will do so because their habit leads to fatal perforations or bleeds from ulcers.

I have to die of something. I have always found that this is said by someone in good health. It is never said by anyone who has already developed a chronic illness, such as heart disease or intractable ulcer disease.

I don't want to be old, anyway. We change our definition of 'old' as we grow older! We would all like to live a long time, but we do not want to be afflicted by the illnesses we see in the elderly. If we take care of ourselves on the way to old age, we will enjoy it much more when we get there. That particularly applies to a good digestion and the ability to eat well and enjoy food.

I'll put on more weight if I stop. That is probably not true for you – although it is true for many smokers. If you have a duodenal ulcer you are probably eating to ease the pain. If you stop smoking and your ulcer heals, you will probably feel like eating less, without feeling too hungry. In any case, stopping smoking will give you back a healthy appetite, so that you will now be enjoying food again, instead of using it as a sort of painkiller! Enjoyment of good food is one of the pleasures of life, and stopping smoking will enhance that pleasure. Even if you do put on weight, the health risks of being a little overweight are less than those of smoking.

I enjoy smoking and don't want to give it up. Are you sure? Is this not an excuse because it sounds better than admitting that you cannot stop? Is there real pleasure in smoking? What exactly is it? Be honest with yourself.

Cigarettes settle my nerves. If I stopped I'd have to take tranquillizers. Smoking *is* a prop, like a baby's dummy. The rituals – the packet, the lighter, the fondling of the cigarette, hooding it with your hands as you light it, holding it in your mouth – are all substitutes for boredom, and even loneliness. But it solves nothing. It certainly does not remove the cause of your stress, and only worsens your long-term health prospects. And if you have an ulcer it will keep it from healing. The resulting continuing pain will *add* to your stress and nerves.

I'll change to a pipe or cigars – they're safer. Not for you they are not! Cigarette smokers who change to pipes or cigars continue to inhale, so that they still have the same levels of nicotine and carbon monoxide in their bloodstream. And they will keep your ulcer going.

I've smoked for 40 years. It's too late to give up. No, it is not. If you stop, within a day or two your ulcer will begin to heal, and within a month your stomach and duodenum will look on the endoscope as if they had never been affected by ulcers. As a bonus you will immediately reduce your risk of a heart attack, and long term, you will greatly reduce your chances of lung cancer. And of course, if you stop today you may just prevent that perforation or bleed that was scheduled for tomorrow! Remember that anyone with an ulcer and who smokes is sitting on a time bomb – no matter how long you have smoked. In fact the longer you have done so, the longer you have had your ulcer, and the more likely you are to meet with catastrophe.

I wish I could stop, but I can't. I've tried everything. Stopping smoking is easy, if you really want to do it. Of course you must put some effort into it yourself. Do not expect someone else to do it for you, and do not rely on some gimmick to help. You must be motivated to stop, and if the last few pages have not motivated you, then you never will be!

Stopping smoking

Getting motivated

What motivates people to stop smoking varies from person to person, and from generation to generation.

Teenagers, for example, care little about long-term health risks. They seem far off, in middle age or old age, and that does not concern them. They may even be attracted to the idea that smoking is a danger. So if you want a teenager not to smoke – and teenagers do get ulcers – then concentrate on the way smoking makes them look and smell. Smoking is smelly and dirty.

It also pollutes the environment and exploits developing world poverty to the benefit of big multinational business. Hundreds of thousands of hectares of good agricultural land is used in Pakistan and Brazil, for example, to grow tobacco for the developed world's pleasure, at the expense of growing food for the poor.

Even worse, the tobacco companies are vigorously promoting their wares to developing world populations, adding lung and ulcer diseases to their already huge burden of ill health. The USA, which is second only to Finland in the restrictions placed on smoking in public, is by far the biggest exporter of cigarettes to others (in Finland now, office workers who wish to smoke have to stand outside at least 15 metres away from their office entrance, which must be quite an ordeal in the Finnish winter).

Where is the teenager who wants to be party to this process of exploitation of poorer people by the rich? Today's students, who have huge worries, both financial and about their future job prospects, and who do develop ulcers, certainly seem to respond to these arguments.

For younger adults, appearance can be the best motivation to stop. Smoking ages people prematurely. Nicotine-induced changes in the skin circulation produce more wrinkles and, in white people, a grey, pasty colour instead of the normal pink complexion. Women suffer more than men from this, mainly because women's magazines constantly show pictures of models with perfect skin. Naturally, they are skilfully touched up, as no one has such a skin. But the image is strongly promoted as a goal. Women who smoke could save themselves the horrendous costs of beauty creams and of their cigarettes, *and* look far better, by giving up smoking. It is strange that the desirable image of men is still that of the Marlboro cowboy, with the craggy lived-in face: the 'laughter lines' are actually produced by smoking. I wonder how many of the original Marlboro men can still laugh – and how many can hardly breathe.

The rapid skin-ageing induced by cigarette smoke is reflected in hormone levels, too. Women smokers have an earlier menopause than non-smokers. Smoking businesswomen who plan to postpone their families until they are in their thirties may well lose out, permanently.

For older men and women the main motivation is health. The statistics on the survival of smokers beyond the age of 60 are terrifying. One-third of men do not live to collect their pensions, and smoking is the main cause of their deaths. If you are male, have an ulcer and smoke, and even this does not convince you to stop, then think of your partner. She will probably be alone for the last 20 to 30 years of her life. Of course she might marry again – hopefully a non-smoker this time!

If you are in your forties or older and you smoke, then it is long odds-on that you already have chronic bronchitis, and your circulation is under attack. If you have an ulcer as well then you are asking for disaster – for three reasons:

1 the nicotine keeps the ulcer active, stopping it from healing. At the least this will keep the pain going. It will also raise the risk of bleeding and perforation, because the risk rises with every day an ulcer exists.
2 if you do bleed from the ulcer the blood loss is likely to be much more severe than normal because the ruptured blood vessel is damaged from the years of abuse and cannot shut off properly.
3 if the ulcer perforates through the stomach wall then you will need emergency surgery. Ask any anaesthetist just how enjoyable it is looking after the lungs of anyone who has been smoking regularly up to the day of the operation! Especially in an emergency, when the patient is already toxic from peritonitis!

How to stop

Now that you are motivated to stop smoking, how do you do it?

First, make sure that your aim is to stop, not just to cut down, then be determined to do so, no matter what. I used to advise people that they had a choice, to cut down gradually, or to stop, once and for all. Now I am convinced that the 'General de Gaulle' method is the best.

The general announced to the whole of France, on television, that he had stopped smoking. From then on he never dared light up in case the press caught him at it and exposed him as a fraud or backslider! Most people could do something similar, in front of friends. In today's antismoking climate you will get much support and sympathy from them.

I advise people to take all their cigarettes, from their pockets, handbags, at home, or wherever, and scrunch them up together. They should then throw them in the bin. They then must resolve never to buy another cigarette, and always immediately say 'no', without thinking about it, to anyone who offers them one. Putting a non-smoking sticker on a car window or even on a window in or near the front door can be an added reinforcement. It helps avoid verbal battles with visitors or friends who may otherwise have lit up.

People contemplating stopping suddenly always fear withdrawal symptoms. They say that they will be irritable, agitated, nervous and sleepless. I have found that people who have had to give up because of serious health reasons, such as recovery from a heart attack or because they have come through a perforation or a major ulcer bleed, hardly ever have withdrawal symptoms. This strongly suggests that they are psychological rather than physical. If you can do something to prevent another visit to the intensive care unit you will be very happy to do it.

So why not stop before the disaster hits you, rather than afterwards? You may not have the chance afterwards! The motive for stopping beforehand is just the same as when you decide to quit while staring at the drip in your arm and the monitor beside your bed.

Second best is to stop gradually. If you take that decision, then the first cigarette to stop if you have an ulcer is the last one at night. Many ulcers are kept going because the stomach keeps producing its acid throughout the night, when there is no food to neutralize it. That last cigarette stimulates the continuing secretion of acid, which prevents any chance of the ulcer beginning to heal.

So if you usually smoke your last cigarette just before sleeping, bring it forward for the first few nights to an hour beforehand. After a week drop *that* cigarette too, and make your last cigarette an hour earlier still. Week by week keep bringing that last cigarette forward until it is in the mid-afternoon – which will usually take about six weeks. A week or two into this plan, start your first cigarette in the day an hour later. Do not keep your cigarettes beside your bed: put them in another room, so that it is a bother to get out of bed to get to them.

Then, week by week, postpone that first morning cigarette by a further hour. So after six weeks your first cigarette of the day meets up with your last! You will find it easiest of all to stop that one.

If you need extra help to stop, carry chewing-gum or nibbles, such as carrot or celery, to chew when you feel the need for a cigarette. Get a friend to support and encourage you, and monitor your progress every day. You can use a graph to do it: some people find it helps to have written proof of their endeavours.

What you should *not* do is use nicotine chewing-gum. Nicotine is after all part of the cause of your ulcer, and it will keep the ulcer open and inflamed – quite the opposite of your main aim. If you use aids to help you stop smoking, like acupuncture and hypnosis, you must realize that they are only a prop. They have no magical properties and cannot provide you with the will to stop. That must come from you.

From the time you reach your planned 'stop' day the break must be complete. You will never buy or accept another cigarette. You will never risk 'just one', even at smoky parties when the drinks are flowing and your resistance is low. Be particularly on the defensive on these occasions. If you accept that one cigarette, you will be back to 20 a day in three weeks.

If you do manage to stop, you will not be on your own. The British are stopping smoking at a rate of a million a year. Only 1 adult in 3 now smokes. All you are doing is joining the sensible majority.

Action on Smoking and Health (ASH)

Now that you have read this far you must already be a non-smoker! How will that change your life? Apart from finding that your ulcer is healing as your craving for nicotine subsides, you will no longer have to put up with the restrictions that smoking places on you. Since 2007 you will have had to leave any public place in the UK to smoke: that may irritate you, but it makes the rest of the public much happier that they don't have to inhale your smoke.

ASH (see Useful addresses) campaigned from 1993 onwards for a smoke-free environment at work, in restaurants, cafes and pubs, in banks and post offices, and in schools. And it continues to campaign today to fight the harm caused by tobacco around the world. It is to ASH's great credit that we now have legislation that outlaws smoking in public places in all the countries of the UK. The benefits are already astonishing. In 2007, the year after the ban started in Ireland, the numbers of heart attacks there fell by nearly 20 per cent, and this was followed by exactly the same results in Scotland, Northern Ireland, Wales and eventually England, as they followed suit.

In the spring of 2011 I asked the doctors in our rural area of Scotland if they had noticed any effect of the ban on their practice workload. It had definitely lessened the doctors' burden of heart attacks and strokes, but they were not so sure about their peptic ulcer cases. Until they looked at their records and found that they had seen fewer episodes of acute peptic ulcer symptoms in their regulars on antiulcer treatments. This is, of course, anecdotal evidence and not published, but it was convincing.

From around 2005 onwards my colleagues had been running smoking cessation clinics, so that they had been tackling tobacco use in the years of the ASH campaign and the antismoking legislation, and they have no doubt that the drop in ulcer cases is directly related to their patients stopping smoking, combined with the steep fall in passive smoke exposure in public places. I would add that over the many years I have looked after patients with peptic ulcers, those who have continued to smoke have never been completely free of their discomfort and more serious symptoms. When you read the benefits of stopping in the following paragraphs, you will understand why smoking is anathema to anyone with a peptic ulcer.

The benefits of stopping smoking

Finally, if you are still finding it difficult to give up, read this list of the benefits of stopping, and let it make your decision for you.

Within 20 minutes of your last cigarette

- your blood pressure falls to normal (smokers' pressures are raised);
- your pulse slows to normal;
- the circulation in your fingers and toes opens up (smoking restricts it);
- the circulation in your stomach and duodenum opens up (starting the healing process if you have an ulcer).

After 8 hours

- the carbon monoxide in the blood and tissues is at the usual vanishingly small level for a non-smoker;
- the oxygen in the blood rises to normal levels.

After 1 day

- your chances of a heart attack fall significantly;
- your chances of an ulcer perforation or bleed fall significantly.

After 2 days

- your senses of taste and smell improve;
- your appetite returns;
- if you have a gastric ulcer there are already visible signs of healing.

After 3 days

- your lungs open out, getting more air deep into them. Breathing is much easier.

After 2 weeks to 3 months

- your gastric ulcer is healed;
- your circulation in general is much improved;
- you can walk further and faster.

After 1 to 9 months

- your chronic cough (admit you have one!) disappears;
- your lungs are cleaner and less prone to infection;
- you have already missed, on average, one episode of duodenal ulcer recurrence.

After 5 years

- your risk of lung cancer drops from 137 to 72 per 1,000;
- you have avoided three or four duodenal ulcer recurrences;
- your gastric ulcer has remained healed.

After 10 years

- your risk of lung cancer drops to 0.12 per 1,000;
- your risks of cancer of the mouth, oesophagus, bladder, kidney and pancreas fall steeply;
- your chances of an ulcer perforation or bleed fall to near zero;
- hopefully, you have forgotten what an ulcer feels like!

It must be worth stopping, not just for your stomach or duodenum's sake, but for everything else, too.

Some thoughts on the smoking ban

I cannot complete this edition of *Coping with Stomach Ulcers* without commenting on one aspect of society that was not present or even predicted in 2002, the year of its previous update – the banning of smoking in public places.

The smoking bans

On 29 March 2004, the Republic of Ireland became the first country in the world to institute an outright ban on smoking in workplaces. Smoking had already been outlawed in public buildings, hospitals, schools, restaurant kitchens and on aircraft and some trains (Intercity trains provided smokers' carriages). On 1 July 2009, the Republic took the further steps of banning in-store tobacco advertising and displays of tobacco products at retail outlets, and adding new controls on tobacco vending machines.

On 26 March 2006, Scotland followed Ireland by prohibiting smoking in enclosed (more than 50 per cent covered) public places, which includes public buildings, workplaces, sports stadiums, bars and restaurants. Hotel guests may still smoke but only in designated smoking bedrooms. My information is that they are few and dingy! Scots law also bans smoking in bus shelters, phone boxes or other shelters that are more than 50 per cent enclosed, and in trucks and vans owned by a company whether or not the driver is the only person inside.

Wales banned smoking in all enclosed public premises and work premises on 2 April 2007, and Northern Ireland followed four weeks later. Their bans include bars, restaurants, offices (even if the smoker is the only person in the office), public buildings, phone boxes and enclosed bus/train shelters.

In England, after a strong but thankfully unsuccessful campaign against the proposed ban, smoking was not allowed in indoor public places, including workplaces, bars, clubs and restaurants, from 1 July 2007. There are more exclusions in the English rules: people can still smoke in some nursing homes, prisons, submarines, offshore oil rigs, and stages/television sets (if needed for the performance). Palaces are also excluded, although members of the House of Commons and the House of Lords agreed to ban all smoking in the Palace of Westminster. So the Royal Family, if they wish, can continue their long love affair with tobacco, which killed the last four monarchs.

The results

So the population of the British Isles, more than 60 million, has taken part in the biggest ever study of the consequences of stopping or reducing smoking. It produced positive health results far faster than anyone imagined. Within a year of each ban, country after country in turn reported significant reductions (of around 20 per cent) in deaths from heart attacks and strokes, and even from lung cancers (the prediction was that they would not fall for many years after the ban).

Naturally, because I was writing this book, I searched the medical literature for any evidence that the incidence of peptic ulcer might also have fallen at the same time. I looked in vain. No one appears to have published any research findings on the subject – possibly because we are already so effective in dealing with peptic ulcer that it is no longer of vital interest. Discussing this point with my fellow GPs, they think this may be the case. They find that, by treating their possible ulcer patients with the standard triple therapy for *Helicobacter*, they no longer have the large numbers of long-term 'chronic stomach patients' on their lists that they had only a decade ago. The public smoking bans, along with the GPs' smoking cessation clinics, may have helped to achieve this, but there are no hard data to confirm this opinion. The only piece of relevant research that I could find on the subject was from the University of Minnesota, where among more than 4,000 smokers and non-smokers aged from 18 to 30 years, the smokers were nearly twice as likely to have numerous ailments, including ulcers, when they were re-examined 7 to 15 years later.

8

Treating ulcers with drugs

On 24 March 1995, the BBC science programme *Tomorrow's World* devoted a few minutes to peptic ulcer. The claim was made that anti-*Helicobacter* treatment would cure far more ulcers, at a far cheaper price and with many fewer problems for ulcer sufferers, than the current treatment with drugs to suppress acid secretion – the H_2 antagonists cimetidine and ranitidine.

The programme encouraged viewers to contact their doctor and demand that they be tested for HP (by the breath test mentioned in Chapter 4). It then proposed that they ask their doctors for anti-HP treatment, and suggested that the programme follow up the results in a year's time.

This was the first television-promoted clinical trial of a new system of treatment for a disease. Sadly, we never heard how many people with an ulcer took up the challenge, and how many of their doctors responded. Doctors do not, in general, take kindly to patients asking them to alter their treatment according to the advice of a television pundit. It is ethically better to base treatments on the findings in each individual case, on the established medical literature on the subject and on the doctor's own experience of similar cases. However, since the programme, the way ulcers are treated has changed, despite the fact that it was in no way a good, controlled scientific comparison of treatments. The numbers involved – it could be several hundred thousand – may make up for this fault.

This chapter gives you, as someone with an ulcer, much more time and many more facts than did *Tomorrow's World*, to help you judge the treatment you are taking or may be offered. It is a review of all the treatments now available, and the reasons behind them.

The principles of ulcer treatment

The treatment of peptic ulcer has four main objectives:

- to ease the ulcer pain;
- to promote healing of the ulcer;
- to prevent ulcers recurring;
- to avoid complications.

Before we consider drug treatment, however, there are some general rules to follow.

The general rules

The first is bed-rest. Now that there are effective ulcer-healing drugs, you no longer need to rest in bed when ulcer pain becomes severe, but it can still help. Before we had drugs like cimetidine and ranitidine, bed-rest and stopping smoking were the only two treatments known to speed up ulcer healing. So if you are going through a bad period, with a lot of pain, and have started on medical treatment, bed-rest for a day or two, but not any longer, is a good idea.

We have already covered stopping smoking. Stopping smoking has been proved to heal gastric ulcers faster and to prevent duodenal ulcers from recurring. Of course, having read this far in the book, you have already stopped!

What you eat matters, but only to the extent that you should avoid foods that you know upset you. It is more important to be positive about food, so rather than thinking about foods to avoid, think about foods you should eat – the varied diet described in Chapter 6. Eat small meals and often, and do not turn to bland, milky diets in the mistaken belief that it will somehow neutralize your 'acid stomach'. It will not.

Avoid drugs that may promote ulcers. Some drugs can irritate the stomach, and this can lead to worsening of an active ulcer. The best known is aspirin. Aspirin has been around for 100 years and is an exceptionally valuable drug for counteracting pain, inflammation and fever. Its usual dose for pain is two or three tablets (of 300 milligrams [mg] each) every 4 hours, and in its usual form this dose irritates the stomach in around 1 in 8 people.

However, there are plenty of aspirin preparations that are relatively 'stomach-friendly'. Most are coated or slow-release preparations. They cost a little more than standard aspirin, but many people find that they can tolerate them better. Your doctor may guide you on what is best for you. If you have had trouble with bleeding after aspirin in the past, however, avoid it. Paracetamol is a good substitute.

As an aside, many people are now taking half or quarter of a standard aspirin a day (75 mg) to protect against heart attack. Most of them have already had a heart attack or are at high risk of heart attacks. This dose of aspirin is very unlikely to irritate the stomach: large trials have shown that it is no worse than a placebo in causing bleeding from the stomach. So you should only stop your daily aspirin if it is actively worsening your symptoms.

NSAIDs – drugs like naproxen, indometacin, ibuprofen and others (see the Appendix for a full list) – usually prescribed for arthritis and long-term muscular pain, are aspirin-like in their ability to irritate the stomach. If you can, avoid them too. However, if you are unfortunate enough to combine an ulcer with arthritis, you may have no option. Your doctor should be able to guide you on the best one for you.

Other 'drugs' that worsen an ulcer include strong tea or coffee, and alcohol. If you are in the throes of acute ulcer pain, avoid them for a while.

Here, one particular group of ulcer-worsening drugs should be mentioned – steroids. Many people must take corticosteroids such as cortisone, prednisone or prednisolone in tablet form for chronic diseases such as severe arthritis or asthma, or after transplant surgery. Unfortunately, one side effect of steroid therapy can be that it masks the signs of peptic ulcers, including perforation. When you are on steroids, if you do develop an ulcer it may be 'silent', so that you have few symptoms. Even a perforation, with its potential for disaster, may initially be symptomless. So if you are taking steroids long term by mouth for any reason, you should be regularly checked for ulcers. And if you feel something going 'vaguely wrong' inside your abdomen speak to your doctor, who will make sure that a possible ulcer and perforation are not missed.

Drug treatments

Drug treatment for ulcers aims to improve the favourable side of the acid/pepsin : mucosal protection equation in the stomach. There are therefore drugs to reduce the acid and pepsin attack on the stomach wall and drugs to improve the mucus protection. More recently, drugs have been introduced to combat *Helicobacter pylori* infection. They deserve a small chapter on their own (see Chapter 9 for the 2011 guidelines on their use).

Most doctors follow well-established steps when they decide on the drug treatment of peptic ulcer, those for duodenal ulcer differing slightly from those for gastric ulcer because of the need to rule out malignancy in the latter.

Duodenal ulcer

Antacids are used first of all to ease the acute symptoms. If endoscopy confirms an ulcer, then a month's treatment with an H_2 antagonist such as cimetidine or ranitidine is given. If the symptoms have by this time subsided, the treatment is stopped. If they are still a bother, the treatment is continued for another month and endoscopy repeated to confirm that the ulcer is still there.

If the ulcer has not healed in that time, another acid-suppressant drug, such as the proton pump inhibitor omeprazole, or the 'mucosal resistance enhancer' or 'cytoprotectant' sucralfate (Antepsin) is given.

The alternative to this strategy is to combine from the beginning the H_2 antagonist with an anti-*Helicobacter* regimen, usually a combination of a bismuth preparation or a proton pump inhibitor with antibiotics. They will be described in detail in the next chapter.

Some duodenal ulcer patients need long-term maintenance treatment to prevent recurrence.

Gastric ulcer

Gastric ulcers are also treated with H_2 antagonists, but before the decision to treat long term is taken, a biopsy must be taken from the edge of the ulcer to make sure that it is not malignant. The treatment then proceeds just as for duodenal ulcer, but the healing process should be confirmed with a repeat endoscopy.

NSAID-related ulcer

Ulcers provoked by NSAIDs usually heal very quickly after they are stopped and an H_2 antagonist is given. If you need to continue with your NSAID, the H_2 antagonist dose may need to be raised and the drug misoprostol added. Misoprostol is a prostaglandin analogue, which counteracts the action of NSAIDs on the stomach, about which there is more later in this chapter. However, the reputation of NSAIDs for causing gastric irritation is probably overblown: there is little good evidence that they often cause severe complications.

Drugs that reduce acid levels

Antacids

Antacids reduce acid levels by reacting with acid already formed inside the stomach to form a neutral substance. Removing the acid gives instant pain relief in most people with ulcer pain. However, in the doses recommended to relieve pain, they do not heal ulcers. Even in the very large doses needed to heal duodenal ulcers, they probably do not even start to heal gastric ulcers. According to family doctor Dipti Amin, the full regime of antacids to cure an ulcer 'requires an intensely obsessional patient and a suitcase in which to carry the drugs home'.

The reason that they are not as effective in gastric ulcers is that they pass from the stomach into the duodenum too quickly for enough acid to be neutralized to make much difference. They only reduce the acid level in the stomach for about 1 hour – and if they are taken only three or four times a day, this leaves 20 or 21 hours a day in which the stomach acid levels are unchanged and free to attack the ulcer.

This is why many proprietary preparations are designed to form foams or gels within the stomach, on the not very well substantiated theory that in this form they will remain in the stomach longer than usual and have more time to neutralize more acid.

The simplest and probably best-known antacid is sodium bicarbonate. It acts very quickly, but in the process of neutralizing the hydrochloric acid in the stomach it produces masses of carbon dioxide gas. The inevitable result is belching and gas and bloating, which can be as uncomfortable as the ulcer. Taking too much sodium bicarbonate can give you systemic alkalosis, in which the body's delicate acid/base balance is tipped too much towards the basic (alkaline). This can be a problem for people with kidney problems. An excess of sodium can also worsen some forms of heart disease and raise an already high blood pressure.

So, on balance, the simplest medicine is not always the best!

The same goes for the next most common antacid – calcium carbonate. Like sodium bicarbonate it also produces carbon dioxide, with the same results. If you take too much, the excess of calcium can lead to high levels in the blood and kidneys, leading to stones and the milk–alkali syndrome described in Chapter 6.

Magnesium-based antacids (they are made up as the oxide, trisilicate and hydroxide) are slower to act than those made with sodium and calcium, but less likely to cause alkali syndrome problems. However, they tend to cause diarrhoea. Aluminium antacids, such as the hydroxide, phosphate or glycinate, are similar in action but cause constipation.

People worry about aluminium in medicines because they fear the well publicized poisonous effects of the metal – the worst being its perceived (and almost certainly erroneous) association with Alzheimer's disease. However, only very tiny amounts of aluminium are absorbed into the body from aluminium antacids, and doses only have to be reduced or the medicine stopped if kidney failure prevents it from being excreted through the urine.

Getting rid of the gas

As explained above, neutralizing acids gives rise to gas, which can be very uncomfortable, causing bloating and pain. Many antacid preparations are therefore mixed with dimethicone, a substance that reduces the surface tension of gas bubbles, allowing them to coalesce and to be expelled more easily.

Alginates

Antacids may also be mixed with alginates, which form a sticky alkaline barrier that protects particularly the lower end of the oesophagus from acid attack.

Antacids and other drugs: interactions

Magnesium and aluminium antacids pose a particular problem for people taking drugs for other illnesses. When in the stomach they bind to drugs such as certain antibiotics; antifungal drugs (prescribed for example for thrush); antimalarials; antiepilepsy drugs such as phenytoin; phenothiazines (for psychiatric disorders such as depression or schizophrenia); penicillamine (for rheumatoid arthritis) and even iron, for anaemia.

When such drugs are bound to antacids they cannot be absorbed into the circulation, so that although swallowed in the normal way they cannot perform the action for which they are prescribed. So infections are not cured, people with epilepsy may start to convulse, depression or schizophrenia may return, arthritis may worsen and anaemia may not respond fast enough. So if you are taking any other prescribed medication, and are thinking of taking an antacid, make sure that your doctor knows and so can advise on one that will not interfere with the prescription drug.

Antacids also cause the urine to become alkaline. Aspirin is excreted faster by the kidneys if the urine is alkaline, so that a normal dose of aspirin is less effective because it lasts a shorter time in the bloodstream. So taking aspirin with an antacid because you feel it will be less of an irritant to your stomach is a mistake: it will not work as well, and you will need higher doses to have the usual effect. Taking a higher dose is more likely to irritate the stomach, which is the effect you wanted to avoid in the first place!

A list of commonly prescribed antacids is given in the Appendix.

H$_2$ antagonists

These include cimetidine (Tagamet), ranitidine (Zantac), nizatidine (Axid) and famotidine (Pepcid). H$_2$ receptors are the structures within the gastric lining cells that, when stimulated by histamine (a chemical 'messenger' in the bloodstream), cause the production of hydrochloric acid by the cell. H$_2$ antagonists occupy the receptors chemically, preventing the action of the messenger upon them, and therefore shutting down the production of acid.

They therefore act on the acid : mucus protection equation earlier in the process than do antacids. Whereas antacids can only neutralize acid after it has formed and been secreted into the stomach, H_2 antagonists prevent its secretion in the first place. This is obviously a more efficient mechanism. The original trials of cimetidine (the first H_2 antagonist) in *duodenal* ulcers showed that it produced healing in around 85 per cent of ulcers within 8 weeks, compared with 30 per cent healing in the placebo-treated control group. However, although the pain of ulcers was relieved in a few days, it needed at least 4 weeks of treatment to heal even the smallest ulcers.

These healing rates are the same for the later H_2 antagonists: ranitidine, nizatidine and famotidine. When the first trials were done, patients were advised to take their tablets five times a day, including a bedtime dose. Now we know that the results are as good with one dose at night or at most twice daily.

Once H_2 antagonist treatment is stopped, unlike with antacids, there is no immediate rebound duodenal ulcer pain; stopping completely does, however, raise the risk of relapse of the ulcer, sometimes quite soon after stopping the drug. So maintenance treatment is started, at a dose of one tablet at night (400 mg cimetidine, 150 mg ranitidine, 150 mg nizatidine or 20 mg famotidine). This brings down the ulcer relapse rate from 80–90 per cent to about 25 per cent in the following year. How long maintenance treatment should be continued is still not completely decided. The current rule is if someone has fewer than two relapses a year, each recurrence should be treated with 8 weeks of H_2 blocker. Four or more relapses a year demand continuous maintenance treatment. Two or three need individual decision making.

In *gastric* ulcer the pain relief is just as rapid as with duodenal ulcers, and cure rates of 75 to 80 per cent have been reported. However, H_2 antagonists do not cure the underlying gastritis described in Chapter 3. Gastric ulcers, like duodenal ulcers, may also relapse after stopping H_2 antagonists, so that maintenance treatment may have to be continued.

As H_2 antagonists can improve the symptoms of stomach cancer, it must not be assumed that a good response to them in a stomach ulcer case rules out malignancy. This reinforces the message that cancer must be excluded by endoscopy in all gastric ulcer cases.

In *oesophagitis*, H_2 antagonists are effective, but the proton pump inhibitors omeprazole and lansoprazole (see next section) probably have the edge over them in effectiveness.

H_2 antagonists are also used in stress ulcers (ulcers that appear in severely ill patients after burns and accidents) and before emergency anaesthesia, particularly before Caesarean births, to avoid the possibility of vomiting and inhaling acid stomach juices.

Side effects

H_2 antagonists are not all alike. They differ in their side effects, and you should be aware of them if you take an H_2 antagonist.

Cimetidine (Tagamet)

This can cause diarrhoea or constipation, rashes, dizziness, tiredness and muscle aches. All are fairly rare and minor, and usually disappear after a few days even if the drug is continued. More important, cimetidine can cause older people to become confused, and it has been reported to cause impotence and a reduced sex drive. Some men have reported that their breasts have swollen. These symptoms are caused by an effect on the liver system for breaking down sex and other hormones, and reverse on stopping treatment.

Cimetidine interferes with the effects of a long list of drugs, because it reduces their absorption from the gut or because of its action in the liver. They include:

- the two antifungals ketoconazole (Nizoral) and itraconazole (Sporanox)
- the anticoagulant warfarin (Marevan)
- the antiasthmatic drug theophylline (Franol, Nuelin, Slo-Phyllin)
- the antiepileptic drugs phenytoin (Epanutin) and carbamazepine (Tegretol)
- the narcotic sedative pethidine, and other opiates
- the group of tricyclic antidepressants
- the local anaesthetic lignocaine
- the antihistamine terfenadine (Triludan)
- the heart-rhythm-correcting drugs amiodarone (Cordarone), flecainide (Tambocor) and quinidine (Kinidin)
- the anticancer drug fluorouracil.

Because it slows the excretion from the kidney of two drugs – the antidiabetic agent metformin and the heart-rhythm-correcting drug procainamide – cimetidine can cause their levels to build up in the blood. This could lead to damagingly low levels of blood sugar in the first case, and an abnormal heart rhythm in the second.

How to deal with all these interactions depends on each case. The doctor may have to alter doses of the other drugs to ensure that the correct effect is being achieved, or it may be decided to switch from cimetidine to another drug with fewer interactions.

The main lesson to be learned from this list is that if you are already on treatment for any other disorder, and your doctor is contemplating treating you for an ulcer, do make sure that you discuss your current treatment before you add cimetidine to it!

Ranitidine (Zantac)

This drug causes a similar list of minor, reversible side effects to that of cimetidine. However, it is much less likely to cause breast tenderness than cimetidine, and it does not appear to cause breast swelling, or impotence or loss of sex drive in men. Patients on cimetidine in whom these symptoms have been distressing have returned to normal on ranitidine. Much less ranitidine than cimetidine gets into the brain, which probably explains why it is much less likely to cause confusion in the elderly.

As ranitidine has much less affinity for liver enzymes than cimetidine it does not interfere with the activity of warfarin, phenytoin or theophylline. Therefore people who develop ulcers while on post-heart-attack anticoagulation, or who have epilepsy or asthma, are usually given ranitidine rather than cimetidine.

Famotidine (Pepcid) and nizatidine (Axid)

These are the newest of the H_2 antagonists. They are more like ranitidine than cimetidine in their side effects. Although famotidine is given in much smaller doses than the others, this does not seem to make its side effects less frequent or severe than those of the other drugs.

The choice – which H_2 antagonist?

How does your doctor choose which H_2 antagonist to prescribe? Given that they have equally beneficial effects, and their side effects, listed above, which look daunting, are actually rare, many doctors feel that they should prescribe the cheapest, which is cimetidine.

However, most would also agree that in young men with frequent ulcer relapses needing long treatment, cimetidine's potential for lowering libido and causing impotence makes ranitidine the choice. In the elderly, too, ranitidine has the advantage that it is much less likely to cause confusion. Famotidine and nizatidine are our third-line choices after cimetidine and ranitidine, mainly because we are a fairly conservative bunch and tend to stick to drugs that we know work and with which we have years of experience.

The proton pump inhibitors

Proton pump inhibitors, such as omeprazole (Losec), lansoprazole (Zoton), esomeprazole (Nexium), pantoprazole (Protium) and rabeprazole (Pariet), act on a different mechanism within the stomach lining cells from H_2 antagonists. The proton pump is the final acid-secreting pathway in the surface of the gastric lining cells. If it is blocked, then no flow of hydrogen ions can escape into the stomach to form the hydrochloric acid. The end result is that the stomach produces no acid at all.

This is a more complete action than H_2 antagonism, as histamine is only one of three mechanisms for stimulating acid production (the others are gastrin secretion and vagus nerve stimulation). H_2 antagonists do not block acid arising from vagus nerve stimulation or gastrin secretion, so some acid, though much less than normal, does pass into the stomach under H_2 antagonism.

Omeprazole (Losec)

In the completely acid-free environment of proton pump inhibition by omeprazole, a dose of 20 mg once daily cures more than 90 per cent of duodenal ulcers in 4 weeks. An 8-week course of the same dose of omeprazole heals 85 to 90 per cent of gastric ulcers.

Omeprazole 20 mg daily is the treatment of choice of the ulcers in oesophagitis: after 4 weeks it heals approximately 80 per cent of them.

It is also the treatment of choice in Zollinger–Ellison syndrome, described in Chapter 2. However, the dose to suppress the huge excess of acid and pepsin activity in such patients is much higher (up to 120 mg per day), and may have to be continued for years.

Omeprazole is also used, like ranitidine, in stress ulcers in acutely ill and burned patients, and in emergency anaesthesia to prevent inhalation of acid vomit. It is being used in trials to see if it will reduce deaths and severe illness from bleeding ulcers.

If you are taking omeprazole, be careful to keep your capsules dry. Omeprazole degenerates if it becomes damp, and the capsules must be kept in a container in which there is a drying agent, usually included in the lid. All the capsules must be taken within 3 months of first opening the container. Omeprazole side effects include diarrhoea and headache, which can be severe. Others are nausea and flatulence, and (paradoxically, in view of the diarrhoea) constipation. Muscle and joint pain, blurred vision, ankle swelling (with fluid), enlarged breasts, loss of taste, blood disorders such as anaemia and loss of white cells, confusion, depression and even hallucinations are all rare side effects.

Its interactions with other drugs include the slowing of the breakdown of the anticoagulant warfarin, the antiepileptic agent phenytoin, and the tranquillizer diazepam. This increases their effects, so that if you are on them and are asked to take omeprazole as well you will probably have to reduce their doses or take them less frequently.

Esomeprazole is virtually identical to omeprazole in its action, effects and side effects; the choice of one or the other is often more linked to the doctor's familiarity with the drug rather than to any advantage one has over the other. Possibly its most common use is in combination with the NSAID naproxen (as Vimovo) for patients with arthritis in whom naproxen alone upsets their stomach. There is a similar preparation combining the NSAID ketoprofen with omeprazole (Axorid), for the same reason.

Lansoprazole (Zoton)

This is the second of the proton pump inhibitors. It is claimed to work faster and more completely than omeprazole – in healthy volunteers 30 mg of lansoprazole made the stomach contents more alkaline more quickly than omeprazole. This is claimed to give faster relief of oesophagitis and stomach ulcer pain than omeprazole. However, it has the same range of side effects as omeprazole. After it was introduced in 1994 it became the second choice for most doctors, and in 2011 it remains so.

Newer proton pump inhibitors

Esomeprazole, pantoprazole and rabeprazole, more recent proton pump inhibitors, are usually prescribed if there have been problems with the two leaders, omeprazole and lansoprazole. They are just as effective and cause just as few side effects as the others, but it is good to have a choice for individual patients who may react badly to one but not another member of the class.

Proton pump inhibitors and stomach cancer

When drugs that suppress all stomach acid, such as omeprazole, were made available, many doctors were worried that they might cause stomach cancer.

The reasoning was clear. We have known since the beginning of the century that most cancers arise in stomachs in which the acid levels have been low for many years. The classical example is pernicious anaemia, in which stomach acid production is faulty, and in which there is a much higher than normal risk of stomach cancer.

It was reasoned that the reduced acidity allowed bacteria, which would otherwise be destroyed by acid, to colonize the stomach. The bacteria targeted as perhaps causing cancer were 'nitrate-reducers', which produce N-nitroso compounds from food. N-nitroso compounds do cause cancer-like changes in experimental conditions and cancers in animals. Add to that the fact that cancers have developed in stomachs from which the acid-producing portion has been removed by surgery, and the fear that acid-abolishing drugs may lead to the same is understandable.

So, when omeprazole was first marketed, its use was restricted to eight weeks, and doctors were warned not to give it on a long-term basis. These rules have now been relaxed. After some years of prescription in millions of people there is no evidence of a link between omeprazole and stomach cancer. Lifelong studies in animals have also failed to show such a link. As long as people taking omeprazole for long periods are regularly monitored for any suspicious change in the stomach, there should be no risk from it or from the other proton pump inhibitors.

Doctors who still wish to play safe, however, tend to prescribe an H_2 antagonist at night, which allows some acid production during the day. This should not only avoid any cancer risk, but should also improve digestion, which needs some acid content after meals.

Prostaglandin analogues

Prostaglandin E_2 is a natural substance that reduces acid secretion, opens up the circulation under the gastric lining cells and stimulates the production of the protective mucus. So a drug acting exactly like prostaglandin E_2 should be beneficial in peptic ulcer.

Misoprostol (Cytotec, Arthrotec, Napratec)

Misoprostol was the first drug with actions similar to those of prostaglandin E_2. Its main use is to prevent stomach and duodenal ulcers in people already receiving NSAID treatment. NSAIDs are antiprostaglandin agents, because prostaglandins forming in inflamed joints are a major cause of pain. One of the side effects of NSAIDs – blocking the formation of prostaglandin E_2 in the stomach – is to promote ulcers in susceptible people. So misoprostol is prescribed to prevent NSAID side effects in the stomach.

However, misoprostol has side effects of its own, which is where life gets complicated! The extra prostaglandin effect often leads to diarrhoea, stomach cramps, nausea and vomiting. It can also cause between-period bleeding in women, and causes rashes and dizziness. It must not be given in pregnancy because it can cause abortion.

It is mainly prescribed in a combination with the NSAID diclofenac (as Arthrotec) or with naproxen (Napratec).

Drugs that improve mucosal resistance

One constant aim in the fight against ulcers has been to produce drugs that improve the mucus protecting the stomach against acid and pepsin attack. Success for a long time was limited, but the research effort did lead to a much better knowledge of the mechanisms of mucus protection, and eventually to worthwhile drugs.

The story starts, however, with very old medicines – liquorice and bismuth. The former has now disappeared from our prescription pads, but I include it for interest and to explain to readers who found it useful why it can no longer be given. Anticholinergic drugs, formerly also used to treat ulcers, have been removed from the prescription list due to side effects.

Liquorice

Some years ago, Dutch doctors found that liquorice helped patients with gastric ulcers, in an undefined way. It did not reduce acid or pepsin secretion, and it was assumed that it changed the nature and increased the volume of the protective mucus within the stomach. Further studies have suggested that liquorice improves the regeneration of stomach mucosal cells around ulcers, and reduces the inflammation around them.

Two medicines were produced out of this research. The first was carbenoxolone (Pyrogastrone), and the second 'deglycyrrhizinated' liquorice (Caved-S).

Carbenoxolone (Pyrogastrone)

Carbenoxolone was given three times a day after meals for 6 weeks, until the ulcer healed. It was mainly used for stomach ulcers, as the healing process depends on a local effect of the drug on the mucus. It remains in the stomach long enough for the contact to be thorough, but it passes too quickly through the duodenum for a local effect to occur there. Carbenoxolone had too many side-effect problems to become a first-line treatment for ulcers and was eventually withdrawn from prescription in the UK, as was deglycyrrhizinated liquorice (Caved-S).

Caved-S was designed to keep the healing effect of liquorice and avoid the serious side effects of carbenoxolone. It was a pleasant liquorice-tasting tablet to be chewed three times a day. Whether it actually helped to cure ulcers is unclear. The good effects on symptoms may have been due to the fact that it also contained aluminium hydroxide, magnesium carbonate and sodium bicarbonate! So it was a prodigious antacid as well as a possible mucus-enhancer.

Bismuth (De-Noltab)

Bismuth preparations have been known for more than 100 years to relieve indigestion, but it is only recently that we have discovered how they work.

The modern preparation, tripotassium dicitratobismuthate (De-Noltab), has been extremely well researched. Taken as one or two tablets in half a glass of water 30 minutes before meals, the bismuth reacts with the stomach acid to form a layer over the whole stomach lining, and particularly over an open ulcer, where it combines with the proteins in the ulcer fluids. This forms a coat that is strongly protective against acid and pepsin digestion. It also stimulates mucus production, and combines with excess pepsin to prevent its digestion of the ulcer base.

The result is a remarkably effective antiulcer preparation that does not affect either acid or pepsin production by the stomach lining cells. Studies have shown that it is as active as cimetidine in healing duodenal and gastric ulcers after 4 to 8 weeks.

However, these are not the only antiulcer effects of bismuth. Bismuth is directly toxic to *Helicobacter pylori*, so that it has become a standard part of the anti-HP treatment described in the next chapter.

Like all active drugs, bismuth has its drawbacks. The liquid form, De-Nol, was eventually removed from prescription because it tasted metallic and smelled like ammonia; the tablets were much more acceptable. People taking De-Noltab should avoid antacids or milk at the same time, as they greatly reduce the effectiveness of bismuth.

The side effects of bismuth treatment include blackening of the teeth, the tongue and the stools. This last is important because it can sometimes be confused with melaena, the black tarry stools of a bleeding ulcer. It makes some people feel sick, and it should not be used by people with chronic kidney disease, as small amounts of absorbed bismuth can build up to a toxic (poisonous) level in the blood if the kidneys cannot cope.

To avoid long-term toxicity, bismuth treatment is not recommended for long-term prevention of ulcers. The maximum recommended treatment is 56 days. Its main use now, however, is to help eradicate HP infection, which is described in the next chapter.

Sucralfate (Antepsin)

The drug with the best credentials as a mucus layer protector is based on neither liquorice nor bismuth. It is sucralfate. An 'alkaline aluminium salt of sucrose octasulphate', in the presence of stomach acid it becomes a sticky paste that adheres to open ulcer surfaces, while remaining a strong antacid. In this it differs from all other antacids, which form gels that lie within the stomach cavity. Sucralfate also binds to pepsin and bile salts, preventing them from coming into contact with the ulcer surface.

In trials it was as effective as cimetidine in healing gastric and duodenal ulcers, and it also gives good relief of symptoms. Because it is virtually unabsorbed into the circulation, it has few side effects, but its aluminium content can cause constipation, and could cause complications in people with kidney failure on dialysis.

It is possible that one reason for the benefit of sucralfate in peptic ulcer is that, as with bismuth, it kills *Helicobacter pylori*. However, that has still to be proved. The current methods for killing *Helicobacter* that *are* proved are described in the next chapter. Unfortunately, the ideal method is still to be found. That *Tomorrow's World* programme may find that it has much to answer for!

9

Getting rid of *Helicobacter pylori*

Most people being offered anti-*Helicobacter* treatment express surprise at the complexity of the drug combination. It is usual for most infections to be given an antibiotic for a few days, and for the infection and the symptoms to clear up. *Helicobacter* treatment is not like that.

This is because HP infections do not follow the usual pattern of infections of, say, the throat, lungs, kidneys or skin. In such infections, the germ hits you, you respond with the symptoms (usually of pain and fever), and a combination of antibiotics and your own immune system throws it off.

Helicobacter has a different plan for its survival. For example, when it first reaches the stomach it does not cause an acute infection, and the body's immune system does not respond with the usual feverish reaction. Most people infected with HP do not know that they carry it. The germ can then happily live on inside the stomach, causing nothing more, in most people, than a chronic gastritis that they know nothing of, because they have no symptoms. Only when an ulcer develops does the infection impinge itself on their consciousness, in the form of pain. This is usually years after the initial infection, and may never even happen.

Second, HP hides itself away from the combined antibiotic and immune system attack by living just under the gastric mucus layer, on the surface of, but not in, the cells themselves. This means that any antibiotic that will kill HP first has to reach it – the antibiotic must be secreted into the mucus in a high enough concentration to kill the bacteria. Many antibiotics can kill *Helicobacter* in culture plates in the laboratory; very few of them can penetrate in high enough concentration into the gastric mucus in living people! In the first trials of anti-HP drugs, most people showed flourishing colonies of the bacteria within a month of so-called eradication.

Third, HP is able to mount considerable resistance to antibiotic challenges. It is extremely impervious to many otherwise useful antibiotics, and can quickly defend itself against others. So it fast became clear from the beginning of our knowledge of the bacterium that it would be useless to attack it with one drug at a time. Combinations would have to be used to ensure its eradication. Of course, this decision posed other problems: the more drugs that are used, the more side effects there will be. This has proved to be so in practice.

Even if an antibiotic gets into the stomach, it may be inactivated by the acid environment. This is the case for many penicillins, which will kill HP in the acid/alkali neutral environment of most body tissues and fluids, but which are ineffective in the acid environment of the stomach.

And the stomach has this annoying habit of emptying every few minutes – so that just as an effective antibiotic is getting to work it is washed away, and the germ gets its reprieve!

Bismuth, in the form of De-Nol, was the first drug to be found effective against HP in people, after it was shown to reduce the recurrence rate of duodenal ulcer more effectively than did the H_2 antagonists. It was then a short step to show that De-Nol had eradicated HP in the patients whose ulcer did not return.

Unfortunately, it soon became clear that when given alone, bismuth only eradicated the germ in 10 to 30 per cent of people. However, bismuth remains important in triple therapy (described below) because it helps prevent HP from developing resistance to the other two drugs. In the bismuth doses used in the triple therapy there are no serious side effects, the only one noticed by its users being a darkening of the stools.

Metronidazole (Flagyl) was initially introduced many years ago for the treatment of thrush. More recently it was shown to be effective in a particular type of gut infection caused by anaerobic bacteria – bacteria that thrive without the need for oxygen. *Helicobacter* is susceptible to it, but soon develops metronidazole resistance if it is prescribed alone.

Tetracycline was developed in the 1940s in the rush of enthusiasm for antibiotics after the success of penicillin. It is still highly successful against bronchial and skin infections. Thankfully, HP is highly susceptible to tetracycline.

Triple therapy

So which antibiotics *do* work against HP? In the first 10 years or so of anti-HP therapy, the choice settled on the combination of three drugs – bismuth, metronidazole and tetracycline (Achromycin, Deteclo, Mysteclin, Sustamycin, Terramycin). This was popularly known by doctors, for obvious reasons, as the triple therapy.

Penicillin (amoxicillin, Amoxil) was sometimes used instead of tetracycline, but the results seemed to be a little better with tetracycline. The choice of tetracycline also avoided the problem, however slight, of penicillin allergy.

However, as experience with the initial triple therapy widened, the guidelines to doctors changed: now we have much more choice of anti-HP treatment, depending largely on how well the patient responds to the first week.

Here are the guidelines in 2011 for UK doctors. Bear with me patiently, because they are complicated! First, the triple therapy using bismuth, as above, is still favoured by some doctors, and continues to work well. But the 2011 edition of the British National Formulary (our 'bible' for prescribing in the NHS) favours a triple therapy that has dropped bismuth as a first-line drug.

We start with a one-week triple therapy of a proton pump inhibitor (usually omeprazole), the antibiotic clarithromycin and either amoxicillin or metronidazole (an antibacterial and antiamoebal drug similar to an antibiotic). If you have recently been prescribed metronidazole or clarithromycin (or a similar type of antibiotic to them) for another infection then amoxicillin is used instead.

This 1 week of triple therapy using any of the combinations above eradicates *Helicobacter pylori* in 85 per cent of cases. There is no need to continue with the proton pump inhibitor afterwards unless the ulcer is very large, when it should be taken for another three weeks. Two weeks of treatment might increase the cure rate further but at the expense of more side effects, so most doctors now limit their anti-HP prescriptions to one week of triple therapy, then stop.

It is vital to use all three components of the triple therapy together, as using only two drugs is much less effective and can lead to the bacterium becoming resistant to them, and its permanent establishment on your stomach lining cells.

If you are already taking an NSAID

Now the scene gets complicated. If your ulcer is thought to be caused by your taking regular doses of an NSAID for chronic pain (as with chronic arthritis or long-standing back pain), then the guidelines for eradicating HP become more complex. If you have stomach problems caused both by the NSAID use and by HP infection (quite a common combination, sadly) then simply giving anti-HP triple therapy as in the previous paragraphs does not often completely rid you of your pain.

It helps you a lot if you can stop the NSAID, but that is not always possible, so you then have the following options after the week of triple therapy:

- You can take a proton pump inhibitor (such as omeprazole) long term, usually at a higher dose than normally recommended, as at the usual dose you can have a 'silent' ulcer returning, which may cause you no symptoms but could still bleed or even perforate.
- You can use a proton pump inhibitor for a further month, then switch to misoprostol long term, although its dose may be limited by colicky pain and diarrhoea.
- You can continue to treat the ulcer with a proton pump inhibitor, but switch your painkilling agent from an NSAID to a type of drug called a cyclooxygenase inhibitor (celecoxib – Celebrex or etoricoxib – Arcoxia).

The coxibs were hugely welcomed when they were introduced in the early 2000s, but have since been implicated in the possible worsening of heart disease, so they are prescribed usually only as a drug of last resort in people with severe pain and continuing ulcers. If you are given one of the coxibs expect to have your heart and blood pressure monitored regularly while taking it.

Keep taking the pills!

The biggest obstacle to the success of triple therapy is when patients forget their daily doses – in medical terms, poor compliance. Not taking all the doses as prescribed is the main reason for failure to cure the ulcer and to eradicate HP. It is also the main reason for the development of resistance to further antibiotic treatment.

It is hard to blame people for poor compliance, because triple therapy involves swallowing a lot of tablets. Bismuth, as De-Noltab, must be taken four times a day, metronidazole three times a day and tetracycline four times a day. This is 11 tablets a day for at least a week.

Not only is the number of tablets a bother, the side effects are annoying, too. Nearly 1 in every 3 people on triple therapy complains of 'significant' side effects – those that are severe enough to complain about. The side effects include malaise, diarrhoea, nausea, a metallic taste and sore mouth, and even pseudomembranous colitis, which is a severe inflammatory reaction in the bowel.

It is very important, therefore, if you are asked to take the triple therapy, that you understand you may have side effects from your drugs, but that you should persist until the end of the course if you can. If you can stick it out, your chances of eradicating HP and getting rid of your ulcer for ever are very high. If you stop in the middle, your ulcer may keep on returning and you may be left with a drug-resistant strain of HP that will not respond to a future course of treatment.

When triple therapy fails, it is usually because the HP strain is resistant to metronidazole – in developed countries the resistance rate is already 10 to 20 per cent. In the developing world, resistance rates as high as 80 per cent have been reported.

Ninety per cent of people with HP respond well to the complete course of triple therapy if the germ is sensitive to all three drugs. However, triple therapy is only 30 to 60 per cent effective in eradicating HP if there is metronidazole resistance – and the high rate of side effects makes it difficult to justify in such circumstances. In the first few years after we started treating ulcers with triple therapy, it was common for specialists to recommend culture of the organisms and testing for resistance before starting therapy. That meant taking biopsies under endoscopy from samples of suspicious-looking stomach wall, or using the 'capsule on a string' approach developed by Dr Perez-Trallero, which was more patient-friendly. However, today's forms of triple therapy seem to cause far fewer side effects and the need for investigations and intrusive examinations is far less than it was. It is years since there was a need for HP culture to test for its resistance in the practices in which I work.

Omeprazole and *Helicobacter*

Helicobacter likes the acid environment inside the stomach. In fact, it likes it so much that when omeprazole is given, and the acid disappears, the HP germs migrate upwards from the last third of the stomach (the antrum, which is usually the most acid area) to the middle of the stomach (the corpus, where some acid remains during omeprazole treatment), to seek out an environment which is as acid as possible.

Why *Helicobacter* should seek out the final remnants of acidity like this is a puzzle. It may be that it is trying to escape immune substances that are more efficient in killing it in less acid conditions; it could be escaping from competition from other bacteria that colonize the stomach only when it is less acid. Whatever the reason, there are fewer *Helicobacter* around in a stomach treated with proton pump inhibitors such as omeprazole.

However, omeprazole alone is not the complete answer. As soon as treatment is stopped, and normal acidity returns to the stomach, the few *Helicobacter* that always survive the low acid conditions migrate back into the antrum and multiply all over again. Within days the normal pattern is resumed.

When treatment does not work

The figures suggest that triple therapy eradicates HP in 90 per cent of patients. For the few people whose HP remains, despite careful adherence to the treatment, some experts advise a quadruple therapy for 1 week. This is the standard triple therapy to which omeprazole 40 mg twice a day is added.

Why take the trouble to get rid of *Helicobacter*?

If all these different regimens seem an awful lot of trouble to go to in order to eradicate a germ in the stomach, then ponder on the possible alternative. That is not just continuing pain for years, on and off, because of recurrent ulcers. It is also the risk of perforation, which eventually happens to 5 per cent of all long-term ulcers, and the risk of bleeding, which occurs in 15 per cent.

For others, such as people with arthritis, the motivation is greater still. They must take NSAIDs to relieve their pain, yet have peptic ulcers because of their NSAIDs. Caught between the pains in their joints if they do not take their NSAIDs and the pain in their stomachs if they do, they are in a quandary.

It was largely resolved by the Glasgow team led by A. S. Taha, who reported in 1995 on 50 long-term NSAID users, 30 of whom were infected with HP. Of these 30, 60 per cent developed gastric erosions and 40 per cent developed ulcers during the study. The corresponding figures for those with no HP were 25 per cent and 15 per cent. The stomach erosions and ulcers were closely linked to HP infections. The authors concluded that anti-HP treatment could well be very important in protecting the stomach and duodenum in NSAID users.

Finally, the evidence that HP promotes cancer of the stomach is becoming stronger. Doctors in Leeds showed that in people with HP and gastritis, a proportion of the stomach lining cells showed precancerous changes (technically called cell proliferation). Within 4 weeks of completing triple therapy to eradicate HP, the changes had decreased – a sign that the cancer risk had receded. In those who continued to harbour HP, the proliferative changes continued to increase.

This is compelling evidence for doing one's best to eradicate HP from the stomach of all people with gastritis and gastric ulcers.

10

Surgery: a last resort

If I had been writing this book in the 1970s, the chapter on surgery would have taken up about half of it. In the days before H_2 antagonists most people with a chronic ulcer were eventually offered surgery. So many operations were performed that some surgeons did nothing else but ulcer surgery.

The surgery itself was still based at that time on the work of surgeons (mainly German) who operated in the early years of the twentieth century. The operations still carried their names – Billroth and Polya were names dear to every medical student, who had to know the differences in nuance between the Billroth I and Billroth II (or Polya) operations. I never did know whether Billroth and Polya were colleagues or rivals!

Thankfully, those days are past. They ended amazingly quickly after the introduction of cimetidine. Once there were good treatments that actually cured ulcers, the surgeons were glad to turn their attentions to other illnesses.

Reasons for surgery

These days the reasons for surgery for ulcers are few. They fall into four categories:

1 failed medical treatment;
2 complications such as perforation, obstruction or haemorrhage;
3 gastric ulcer if there is any suspicion of cancer;
4 an ulcer at the site of an old surgical join line or anastomosis.

It is very rare for medical treatment to fail nowadays. We do not consider treatment a failure until a patient has had at least 6 months of medical treatment with drugs such as cimetidine or ranitidine.

Occasionally, thankfully much less often than in the past, someone who has had a duodenal ulcer for years has been left with a scar that narrows the entry to the duodenum. This pyloric stenosis may have to be widened if the obstructive symptoms (mainly vomiting of food eaten hours or even days before) are interfering with the person's quality of life.

Perforations must be treated as an emergency. This usually means simple oversewing of the perforation site – the hole – and letting the patient recover before taking stock of his condition. For most patients, medical treatment is all that is needed afterwards. Now that we have ulcer-curing drugs only a very few need further surgery later.

Other than these cases, no one has an operation today unless the surgeon has seen an active ulcer under endoscopy. If there is continuing dyspepsia without an ulcer being present, this is a strong sign of nervous dyspepsia – for which an operation can spell disaster. It would solve nothing, and confirm the person in his or her neurosis.

Operations for ulcer

Partial gastrectomy

In the past, surgeons sought to remove most of the acid-producing areas of the stomach, in an operation called partial gastrectomy. This left the person with a stomach about a third of the normal size. Usually the acid problem was solved (about 15 per cent had various complications afterwards), but it was necessary to eat regular small meals from then on. However, most patients thought this preferable to their previous life of constant pain.

Proximal gastric vagotomy

Today, if surgery is unavoidable, surgeons try not to cut into the stomach at all. They prefer instead to cut part of the vagus nerve as it passes to the stomach, thereby decreasing considerably the main nervous stimulus to acid secretion. It involves careful dissection and teasing out of the nerve. This operation, called proximal gastric vagotomy (PGV), cuts only the nerves leading to the area of stomach that produces the bulk of the acid, and leaves intact the nerves that control the coordination of the stomach movement and the passage of its contents towards the duodenum.

The advantages of PGV over partial gastrectomy are that it has a very low mortality rate and very few side effects. However, the ulcer recurrence rate is relatively high. It is hoped that by the time an ulcer has had time to recur in such people, one of the medical treatments, such as the combination of omeprazole and triple therapy, will have been successful.

Post-partial gastrectomy syndromes

A measure of the modern medical treatments for ulcers is that partial gastrectomies have gone from being the most common abdominal operation, after appendicectomy, to one of the rarest. However, some readers of this book will have had a partial gastrectomy, so for them a paragraph or two on their unwanted after-surgery effects and how to manage them may be appropriate.

Small stomach syndrome With this you start to feel full halfway through a normal-sized meal. It is usually best dealt with by eating little and often.

Dumping syndrome Along with a full feeling, you feel suddenly very weak and faint while eating. It usually occurs only when sitting up or standing, and is probably caused by over-distension of the small bowel just beyond the duodenum, the jejunum. It gradually disappears after the operation. While it is happening, it is best to eat dry meals with very little fluid, and to lie down while eating or just after a meal.

Hypoglycaemia Attacks of low blood sugar occur about 2 hours after eating, and symptoms include dizziness, light-headedness, sweating, palpitations and sometimes confusion. It is caused by the too-sudden absorption from the small intestine of large amounts of sugar. This in turn leads to over-release of insulin from the pancreas, which in turn again leads to a much lower blood sugar than normal. The low blood sugar then gives rise to the symptoms. The answer is to eat little and often – small meals low in sugar content. If symptoms start, swallow some sugar at once.

Bilious vomiting Many people vomit small amounts of bile after surgery. It usually settles on its own. Sometimes it is helped by lying on the left side to drain a loop of bowel left by the operation.

Recurring dyspepsia If the pain returns after surgery, it is usually caused by an ulcer at the site of the surgical junction of the two parts of the stomach – the anastomosis. This must be diagnosed by endoscopy and treated urgently with medicine, such as an H_2 antagonist, which is continued for at least a year. If that fails, a further operation is needed. If no ulcer is seen, then the diagnosis is nervous dyspepsia, and appropriate medical treatment is started.

Diarrhoea Many people have looser motions after their operation. This usually responds to constipating drugs such as dihydro-codeine. Some people who have had an ulcer even welcome their looser stools, as they have been used to constipation all their lives!

Anaemia In some people, the lack of acid in the stomach and the hurry of food through the intestine reduces the absorption of iron, and anaemia results. They respond well to simple iron tablets, which are absorbed normally.

Bone problems Very rarely, calcium absorption is disturbed after operation, and the bones can become weaker, leading to fractures. Blood tests will confirm the lack of calcium, which can be replaced with calcium tablets by mouth.

Cancer Cancer at the site of anastomosis is a slight risk, but usually only 10 years or more after the surgery. Any deterioration in health, particularly loss of appetite and weight, should be reported to your doctor.

11

The future: getting rid of *Helicobacter* – and ulcers – worldwide?

Fifty years ago, the link between atrophic gastritis and stomach cancer was made, and the study of gastritis became a priority for researchers all over the world for clues to the cause of stomach cancer.

These studies then discovered links between poor social conditions, gastritis, peptic ulcers, pernicious anaemia and stomach cancer. The links were the same the world over, but the common factor in them all was a mystery until Dr Marshall's discovery of the strange curved bacterium in 1982.

Since then, the increase in our knowledge of *Helicobacter pylori* has been astonishing. Thousands of papers about it have been produced, and it is clear that it is the main cause of one of the biggest epidemics that the world has ever known – touching every nation and every ethnic group.

It is established that first comes HP infection – early in life in the developing world, later in the developed world. Then comes gastritis and, after a short time in a substantial minority of people, gastric or duodenal ulcer. After a longer time, in a much smaller minority, it causes stomach cancer.

Once it is realized that HP is an infectious disease, it should be treated like one. It is more vulnerable to treatment than other diseases we have conquered, such as smallpox. It can be treated successfully and it only seems to survive within humans – so why do we not tackle it appropriately?

This idea has occurred to the experts. Experts in HP, such as Professor David Graham of Houston, Texas, proposed as long ago as the 1990s that it is really a public health problem and should be eliminated from the world's populations, just as smallpox has been eliminated.

One way to do so, he suggests, is to improve standards of living and sanitation worldwide. Another is to use breath tests to detect carriers in the 'healthy' population and give them antibiotics to eradicate their HP. A third is to develop vaccines. 'We could start', he writes, 'in countries with First World economies and "developing world stomachs", like Japan, Saudi Arabia and Korea, where HP infection and gastric cancer are rife.'

HP is an infection, and an infection can be eradicated. If it were, then the twin scourges of peptic ulcers and stomach cancers would be over, for ever. Millions of lives would be saved worldwide. The tools needed to begin an eradication programme are already available. What is now needed is a cost-effective plan to accomplish it.

In the summer of 2002, in my first update of this book, I wrote that 'there are signs that we are winning in the battle against peptic ulcers'. Dr N. J. Talley, together with colleagues at the University of Sydney, had just reported on his hospital's records on ulcers and *Helicobacter* infection among patients seen in 1990, 1994 and 1998. They showed that peptic ulcers were disappearing fast. In 1994, 22 per cent of the patients they were investigating had ulcers. By 1998 this figure had dropped to 13 per cent, and the drop was almost entirely in stomach ulcers and a corresponding fall in *Helicobacter* infections.

However, there was a catch. Several research groups had linked the increasing use of the group of painkillers and antiarthritic drugs known as NSAIDs with stomach ulcers. The best known is aspirin, but naproxen, indometacin and ibuprofen are also household names in the NSAID group. Hong Kong gastroenterologist F. K. L. Chan proposed in 2001 that if your doctor is thinking of giving you these drugs, you should be first tested for *Helicobacter*, and given triple therapy to eradicate it if the test is positive. He added that you should have antiulcer drugs if you need long-term treatment with NSAIDs. 'That may', he wrote, 'even apply to the small dose of aspirin many people take to prevent heart attacks.' This may be a bit extreme, but it shows that we should take particular care in deciding how to treat everyday aches and pains.

NSAIDs are now widely available over the pharmacy counter without prescription. They are not as innocent as they seem. When Dr M. Tsokos of Hamburg University studied the post-mortem examinations of young adults who had died unexpectedly and suddenly, he found seven cases in a year in which the death was linked with stomach ulcers provoked by an NSAID. The three drugs involved were ibuprofen, diclofenac and ketoprofen, all easily obtainable. No other drugs were involved. He fears that we underestimate the numbers of young adults who suffer severe illness or even die from ulcers because they do not know of the potential harm to be done by NSAIDs.

Finally, if you are to get rid of your *Helicobacter*, what is the guarantee you will not catch it again? Sadly, there is no guarantee. Dr M. Seo of Fukuoka University, Japan, followed 107 people with proven ulcers for 2 years after having different treatments to eradicate *Helicobacter*. In ten of them, the *Helicobacter* infection returned in that time. It turned out that in seven of these, the combination of drugs used had not been enough to kill off all the germs, and that the reinfection was in fact regrowth of the survivors of the original bacteria. He stressed (in a 2002 edition of the *Journal of Clinical Gastroenterology*) that doctors must use the most effective combination to eradicate the germ, even if it means higher drug costs. That means at least three drugs at a time, as in the triple therapy described in Chapter 9.

Happily, in 2011, looking back on that 2002 update, I can write with confidence that peptic ulcers, in the stomach and the duodenum, are continuing to cause fewer problems. We GPs are seeing fewer cases than in 2002, and we are more successful in treating them, with higher cure rates and fewer recurrences. I am sure, especially after discussing this with my colleagues, that this is largely because the newer triple regimen for eliminating HP infections is more efficient, and our patients are more knowledgeable about it and understand why they need to follow our instructions to the letter. They are also aware of the dangers of NSAID use, and come to us earlier than ever before when they have problems with them. We did not need to implement Dr Chan's proposal to test for *Helicobacter* in everyone we were going to give an NSAID, but we always discuss with them beforehand the possibility of peptic ulcer, so that they know what they might expect. That seems to have been enough.

So I remain optimistic that we are beating peptic ulcers. We have progressed in our understanding and our management of them since the first edition of this book, and the result has been a steep drop in the numbers of emergency admissions to hospital for bleeding and perforating ulcers. I am certain that this trend will continue. As it has been maintained over years in which people have had much greater access to NSAIDs through pharmacies and supermarkets, and now over the internet, it surely means that our messages are getting through. I look forward to the time when no one needs to read this book!

Appendix

Drugs used in the treatment of ulcers

Many of these former prescription-only drugs are now sold over the counter in pharmacies. They have many different brand names. If you wish to use them, please talk them over with your pharmacist, who is fully trained to give you comprehensive advice.

Antacids

This list of drugs is by no means complete – which shows how big the antacid market is, and perhaps that none of them is ideal! Most contain a mixture of antacids, and many also contain alginate or dimethicone. Some have other actions, but they are included here because acid neutralization is their main action.

- Acidex
- Actonorm
- Algicon
- Altacite
- Alu-cap
- Aludrox
- aluminium hydroxide
- Asilone
- Carbellon
- Gastrocote
- Gaviscon
- Gelusil
- hydrotalcite
- Kolanticon
- Maalox
- Mucogel
- Nulacin
- Peptac
- Simeticone
- Topal

Cytoprotectants

These drugs are thought to act by improving the quality and/or amount of the protective gastric mucus. They differ mainly in their side effects, although there is better evidence for cytoprotection by sucralfate than for the bismuthate, the main action of which is probably as an anti-*Helicobacter* agent.

- sucralfate (Antepsin)
- tripotassium dicitratobismuthate (De-Noltab)

H₂ antagonists

These drugs have similar actions on the stomach – they all greatly reduce acid secretion. They differ in their side effects, in that cimetidine has extra effects on the liver and brain that are much less obvious with, for example, ranitidine. The side-effect profiles of all four currently used H_2 antagonists are well known, now that they have all been used for many years in millions of people.

- nizatidine (Axid)
- cimetidine (Tagamet)
- famotidine (Pepcid)
- ranitidine (Zantac)

Proton pump inhibitors

These drugs suppress all acid secretion. Designed as once-a-day drugs, they are probably equally effective. As omeprazole was the first, it is still the usual drug of first choice, but the others are equally effective and have similarly few and minor side effects. Often it is a matter of the GP's preference, after experience with the different drugs, which you are likely to be prescribed. Cost to the NHS, of course, does come into the choice, too.

- omeprazole (Losec)
- esomeprazole (Nexium)
- rabeprazole (Pariet)
- pantoprazole (Protium)
- lansoprazole (Zoton)

Anti-*Helicobacter* treatments

The main regimens are probably equally effective, provided the whole course is taken as advised. The main cause for failure is missing out on doses, or stopping treatment too early. About one-third of people taking anti-*Helicobacter* treatment have side effects, but if they can stick to the treatment despite the side effects, they can virtually guarantee successful eradication of HP. The details of each treatment are given in Chapter 9.

Triple therapy Any combination of one of the five proton pump inhibitors with two of these three antibacterial agents – amoxicillin, clarithromycin and metronidazole.

The internet

The internet has changed the way we access information on health beyond anything we could have dreamed of in 2002, when I last updated this book – but not always in a helpful or beneficial way. It is not easy to judge, without having medical training, the merits and faults of articles presented on the 'net'.

Searching it in 2011, I found several articles on peptic ulcer, some purportedly by doctors, that were promoting (often with great subtlety) the authors' own products and forms of diet, which have not been put to scientific scrutiny and which dismissed or failed to mention the huge advances in ulcer management in the last 10 years or so. They promote such 'cures' as cabbage juice, chilli peppers, vitamin supplements and lifestyle changes. They may or may not have some merit – I have no way of knowing whether or not they do, because the scientifically controlled trials of such approaches have not been published. So my advice about them is to be wary: please talk over your problems with your doctor, rather than depend on an internet blog that could be at least irrelevant to you, and at most even dangerous.

However, there are excellent academic sites from which you can cull unbiased information that is helpful: one I recommend is <http://www.patient.co.uk/doctor/Peptic-Ulcer-Disease.htm>. It has been updated regularly. It shows the figures for peptic ulcer in the population in 2010, which are strikingly different from those just 10 years ago.

For example, now, *Helicobacter pylori* infection is implicated in about 95 per cent of duodenal ulcers and 80 per cent of gastric ulcers. About 4 in 10 of the whole population, men and women, have dyspepsia at least once a year: 1 in 20 sees their doctor for it, and 1 in 100, presumably mostly those who have not responded to anti-*Helicobacter* therapy or who have features that might lead their doctor to decide to rule out cancer, is referred for endoscopy.

Of this 1 per cent of the population, about 40 per cent have non-ulcer dyspepsia (what used to be called nervous dyspepsia), around the same number has acid reflux oesophagitis, and only 1 in 8 has an ulcer. Two per cent of patients referred for endoscopy turn out to have gastric cancer, and 1 per cent oesophageal cancer.

Before the discovery of *Helicobacter*, and our almost universal use of triple therapy against it, duodenal ulcer was ten times more common in men than in women and there were three men to every two women with gastric ulcer. Now, there are far fewer cases in both sexes, largely because of *Helicobacter pylori* eradication, and the sex incidence is more even. It used to be claimed that over a lifetime around 12 in every 100 of us, males more than females, would develop a peptic ulcer of either type. Today, it is thought that the numbers are fewer, by how much we really do not know, and that the excess of ulcers in men has gone. Now, men and women have roughly the same, much smaller risk of developing an ulcer than before. Our best guess is that, in a lifetime, about 1 in 10 of us, men and women, may develop an ulcer, and that about 4 in 10 of us will have non-ulcer dyspepsia around once a year, only a very few cases of which are actually caused by ulcer. Our 'wars' on *Helicobacter* and on tobacco, and our understanding of the problems produced by NSAIDs, appear to have worked extremely well in reducing peptic ulcer rates and their complications. I'm sure that this will continue.

Glossary

Alginate A seaweed-derived preparation that aims to protect the mucosa from acid and pepsin attack.

Antacid A drug that neutralizes acid already secreted into the stomach by the parietal cells.

Antibacterial agent A drug that attacks bacteria: it can be synthetic, like metronidazole, or made from the products of other microscopic organisms, usually fungi, like penicillin.

Antibiotic An antibacterial drug, such as penicillin and tetracycline, made from the products of other microorganisms.

Antrum The part of the stomach containing the bulk of the acid-producing parietal cells.

Cardia The junction between the oesophagus and the stomach.

Corpus The main body of the stomach.

Cytoprotectant A drug, such as sucralfate, thought to augment the protection given by the gastric mucus against acid and pepsin attack.

Dimethicone A surface tension-reducing agent to relieve flatulence, while protecting the mucosa.

Duodenal cap Part of the duodenum seen on X-ray, which may often show scarring from old or current ulceration.

Duodenum The section of small bowel into which the stomach empties.

Endoscopy The use of a flexible fibre-optic tube to see directly into the oesophagus, stomach and duodenum.

Flagellae Fine, hair-like appendages on *Helicobacter pylori*. Thought to help them swim in the gastric mucus, or perhaps to allow them to adhere to the surface of cells.

Gastric Pertaining to the stomach.

Gastrin A hormone produced in the bowel wall and pancreas that causes parietal cells to secrete acid.

H$_2$ antagonist A drug, such as cimetidine and ranitidine, that blocks the histamine-stimulated secretion of acid by parietal cells. It does not block all acid secretion.

Helicobacter pylori A curved, flagellated bacterium, thought to thrive only in the human stomach, that causes gastritis, gastric and duodenal ulcer and probably gastric cancer.

Hiatus hernia A condition in which part of the stomach has risen above the diaphragm. It leads to oesophagitis and oesophageal ulceration. Symptoms include heartburn.

Jejunum The part of the small bowel after the duodenum.

Metaplasia A change in a tissue towards a tissue of another type. It occurs in duodenal ulcer, which arises in a patch of duodenal mucosa that has changed into gastric type.

Mucosa The layer of cells lining the stomach. It is responsible for the secretion of acid and pepsin and also of mucus. The balance is a fine one, and when disturbed in favour of the former, leads to gastritis and ulcer.

Mucus The thick gelatinous fluid secreted by the stomach mucosa to protect itself against acid and pepsin attack.

Oesophagitis Inflammation of the oesophagus, usually from acid reflux caused by hiatus hernia. It can lead to ulceration of the oesophagus.

Oesophagus The gullet – from the throat to the diaphragm.

Parietal cells The cells in the gastric mucosa that secrete acid. Also called oxyntic cells.

Partial gastrectomy An operation to remove the acid-secreting area of the stomach.

Pepsin The digestive juice secreted, along with acid, in the stomach which begins the digestion of proteins in food.

Proliferation Abnormal multiplication of cells seen in some chronic gastric ulcers infected by *Helicobacter pylori*. Thought to be a pre-cancerous process.

Proton pump inhibitor A drug, like omeprazole and lansoprazole, that blocks all acid production by the parietal cells.

Pyloric stenosis Narrowing of the pylorus by scarring from old duodenal ulcers. It can cause obstruction of the flow of food from the stomach into the duodenum.

Pylorus The junction between stomach and duodenum.

Stoma A new opening between the stomach and the small intestine at a partial gastrectomy operation. Often the site of ulcers after operation.

Ulcer A break in the normal continuity of the gastric or duodenal mucosa, leading to an open sore.

Vagotomy An operation to cut the vagus nerve, thereby reducing acid secretion.

Vagus nerve The nerve (leading directly from the brain) controlling gastric secretion of acid and pepsin.

Useful addresses

Action on Smoking and Health (ASH)
First Floor, 144–145 Shoreditch High Street
London E1 6JE
Tel.: 020 7739 5902
Website: www.ash.org.uk

The Society of Teachers of the Alexander Technique
First Floor, Linton House
39–51 Highgate Road
London NW5 1RS
Tel.: 020 7482 5135
Website: www.stat.org.uk

www.patient.co.uk/doctor/Peptic-Ulcer-Disease.htm
A website full of useful and unbiased information about all aspects of
peptic ulcer disease.

Index